— THE —
Acid
WATCHER
Diet

THE
Acid
WATCHER
Diet

A 28-DAY REFLUX PREVENTION
AND HEALING PROGRAM

Jonathan Aviv, MD, FACS

HARMONY

BOOKS · NEW YORK

Published in the United States by Harmony Books, an imprint of the Crown Publishing Group, a division of Penguin Random House LLC, New York.
crownpublishing.com

Harmony Books is a registered trademark, and the Circle colophon is a trademark of Penguin Random House LLC.

A previous edition of this work was self-published in the United States in different form as *Killing Me Softly from Inside* by CreateSpace Independent Publishing Platform, North Charleston, SC, in 2014.

Library of Congress Cataloging-in-Publication Data
Names: Aviv, Jonathan, author.
Title: The acid watcher diet: a 28-day reflux prevention and healing program / Jonathan Aviv, MD, FACS.
Description: First edition. | New York: Harmony, 2017 | Includes index.
Identifiers: LCCN 2016027557| ISBN 9781101905586 (paperback) | ISBN 9781101905593 (ebook)
Subjects: LCSH: Gastroesophageal reflux—Popular works. | Gastroesophageal reflux—Prevention. | BISAC: MEDICAL / Nutrition. | HEALTH & FITNESS / Diseases.
Classification: LCC RC815.7 .A95 2017 | DDC 616.3/24—dc23
LC record available at https://lccn.loc.gov/2016027557.

ISBN 978-1-101-90558-6
Ebook ISBN 978-1-101-90559-3

PRINTED IN THE UNITED STATES OF AMERICA

Illustrations by Anna Karbashyan
Cover design by Jennifer Carrow

20 19 18 17 16 15 14 13 12 11

First Edition

To Caleigh, Nikki, and Blake for their love and support

Quality is not an act, it is a habit.

—ARISTOTLE

Contents

PART III

THE 28-DAY BLUEPRINT FOR REDUCING ACID DAMAGE, REVVING UP METABOLISM, AND STAYING HEALTHY FOR LIFE

INTRODUCTION

Amber, a thirty-seven-year-old work-at-home mom, is very worried because for the past seven months she has felt a lumplike sensation in her throat. She has difficulty swallowing solid foods, and sometimes even pills seem to get stuck in her throat. Her voice is strained, occasionally raspy, and she feels thick mucus in her throat and a postnasal drip. She is constantly clearing her throat, day and night. She saw her primary doctor, who started her on some allergy medications, but her complaints persisted.

Amber confided her concerns to a friend who had similar symptoms and suggested that Amber see an ear, nose, and throat (ENT) doctor. She was ultimately referred to me, and when I saw Amber in my office I first asked her about her diet and lifestyle. She started every morning with the first of three cups of coffee, and a glass of either orange juice or grapefruit juice. Lunch typically was some sort of tomato-based salad with a lemon-vinaigrette dressing. Family dinner during the workweek was at 6:30 p.m., when she had one or two glasses of wine at dinner. Generally, around 10:00 p.m. she had a snack of a chocolate square or two with a cup of herbal tea.

Examination of her throat with a small camera showed that the normally thin, vibrating vocal cords were swollen like kielbasa and there was a great deal of swelling in the back of the larynx, in the area where the esophagus begins.

As the clinical director of the Voice and Swallowing Center at ENT and Allergy Associates in New York City, I see patients like Amber every day: people who have acid reflux disease but who break the mold for what used to be considered the typical acid-damaged individual. (If you've ever seen Alka-Seltzer commercials from the 1970s and 1980s, you know what I mean—to have acid reflux, you had to be a white, overweight, middle-aged man who had just overindulged in burgers, pizza, and meatballs and was complaining of heartburn.) Today, acid damage is a more universal problem; it doesn't just manifest itself in heartburn, and it afflicts people of all races and ages, including the very young. It keeps both men and women up at night and clearing their throats all day.

What's also changed is the definition of acid damage. You were once thought to be dealing with excess acid only if you demonstrated the classic symptom of heartburn, which, despite its name, is caused by the regurgitation of stomach acid into its adjacent organ to the north, the esophagus, not the heart. But as you'll discover in *The Acid Watcher Diet,* this is a narrow, misleading, and in some instances dangerous definition. In addition to heartburn, the symptoms of acid damage can include the following:

- hoarseness
- a chronic, nagging cough
- a sore throat that appears out of nowhere
- a feeling of a lump being stuck in your throat
- postnasal drip
- allergies
- shortness of breath
- abdominal bloating

These symptoms may be present *with* or *without* heartburn or indigestion. For this reason, millions of people with acid reflux are going undiagnosed—and putting themselves at risk of long-term side effects and potentially deadly diseases, including cancer.

. . .

More alarming than the evolving demographic of the acid-injured, the expanding list of symptoms, and the seriousness of potential consequences is the sheer number of people affected: At least sixty million Americans have acid reflux disease—the most common of acid-related disorders. This is more than the number of people affected by heart disease, diabetes, and celiac disease. And a growing number are succumbing to esophageal cancer—the most extreme manifestation of acid damage. Esophageal cancer has seen a 650-fold increase since the 1970s and is poised to replace colon cancer as the second most common cancer in the United States. Interestingly, the rise in esophageal cancer occurred over the same period that the battle against other forms of cancer—including breast cancer—had made great strides.

There are a number of possible contributing factors to the astounding increase in cases of esophageal cancer:

- Delayed treatment: Too many people tolerate the inconvenience of reflux-related symptoms for years, letting acid damage go unchecked. Because of a misunderstanding of symptoms, they may not even know that acid is to blame. For example, did you know that acid reflux disease is the most common nonlung, nonallergy cause of chronic cough?

- Incorrect treatment: When it comes to excess acid, solutions based on pseudoscience abound, including the use of pH value (acidic versus alkaline) to distinguish healthy from nonhealthy foods. Some of these supposed solutions—especially dietary—not only are ineffective but can dangerously worsen acid damage and pave the way for precancerous conditions to develop.

- Missed diagnoses: Many healthcare professionals are often perplexed by reflux symptoms. Are your symptoms due to allergies or a lung or digestive issue, and to which type of doctor should you be sent first? Many of my patients have seen multiple doctors and been seeking the right treatment for years before they land in my office. Meanwhile, their acid reflux has continued on unchecked.

- Misuse of and/or overreliance on acid-blocking medications: A significant percentage of people who've been prescribed antacid medication do not follow the medication's instructions to a T, a strict requirement for it to be fully effective. The other issue with medications such as proton pump inhibitors (PPIs), which can play a critical role in treating acid reflux when prescribed and taken correctly, is that many people continue to ingest acidic foods and beverages, thereby letting the acid damage continue despite a lessening of symptoms.

Still, these issues don't get to the origin of acid damage; they don't answer the question of why so many of us are plagued by acid reflux and its attendant symptoms in the first place. To answer that, we have to look to the foods and beverages we eat and drink every day. That's where we'll find the one component that's doing all the damage: dietary acid. Whether you know it or not, dietary acid is lurking in many of the foods we consume and presume to be harmless.

And this brings me to why I've written this book: we are at a critical tipping point concerning acid-related disease. We can no longer continue to ingest with every meal the excess of acid that our foods and beverages contain. Nor can we continue to indulge in foods that contain chemicals that alter the natural antacid protective barriers that our bodies already have in place. And we can't settle for subpar or outdated treatment, missed diagnoses, and misused or overused medications. That is, unless we want to deal with the consequence of losing a growing number of our loved ones to a serious and devastating form of cancer—the five-year survival rate of advanced-stage (when it's usually detected) esophageal cancer is only 10 to 15 percent. Practically speaking, most people diagnosed with advanced-stage esophageal cancer will not live longer than one year past diagnosis. According to *A Cancer Journal for Clinicians,* in 2016 it is estimated that there will be 16,900 new cases, with 15,690 deaths.

The Solution: Putting an End to Acid Damage

If you're like most of my patients, you are experiencing a constellation of problems directly and indirectly related to acid reflux and your first order of business is to feel better, and *The Acid Watcher Diet* will help you achieve this. It used to be that the only acid that concerned doctors was the refluxed variety that went *up* from the stomach into the esophagus, and the mission was to alleviate the discomfort that comes with it. Now we know that the problem is not just the acid that goes up into the esophagus from your stomach, but the acid that comes *down* the esophagus when you ingest certain foods and beverages. We also know that this two-way infusion has destructive potential way beyond the discomfort of the burn, which is typically a precursor and an indicator of other problems that start with the food choices you make. When you follow the plan featured in the pages ahead, you will learn how to finally stop the flood of acid that comes in with the foods and beverages you consume, and the gastric acid that refluxes up from your stomach into delicate tissues of the esophagus.

At the heart of this book is the 28-day program I've created to teach you how to use food as the ultimate medicine by identifying what foods to avoid (to stop the damage) and what foods to eat (to promote healing). This program is the result of eight years of work and has evolved from basic food lists into a structured, two-phase program featuring weeks' worth of menu plans and over seventy recipes. More than four thousand of my patients have tested the various iterations of the Acid Watcher Diet and now, as a reader of this book, you are getting the most evolved version yet.

Raising awareness about the sources of dietary acid and recognizing the symptoms of acid reflux beyond heartburn could save your life. The following quiz will provide you with a glimpse at some of these symptoms (to be covered in much greater detail in the pages to come) and help identify your starting point.

QUIZ: Do You Have Acid Damage?

Within the last month, how did the following problems affect you?
(0 = no problem; 5 = severe problem):

1.	Hoarseness or problem with voice	0 1 2 3 4 5
2.	Clearing your throat	0 1 2 3 4 5
3.	Excess throat mucus or postnasal drip	0 1 2 3 4 5
4.	Difficulty swallowing food, liquids, or pills	0 1 2 3 4 5
5.	Coughing after you eat or after lying down	0 1 2 3 4 5
6.	Breathing difficulties or choking episodes	0 1 2 3 4 5
7.	Troublesome or annoying cough	0 1 2 3 4 5
8.	Something sticking in throat or lump in throat	0 1 2 3 4 5
9.	Heartburn, chest pain, indigestion	0 1 2 3 4 5

TOTAL (RSI*) _____

*Reflux Symptom Index (RSI). A score of greater than 13 strongly suggests that the patient has throatburn reflux. A single severe symptom does not a diagnosis make; however, it does suggest that inflammation is present and can be alleviated by following the diet featured in this book.

Reprinted from *Journal of Voice,* 16(2), Belafsky, P.C., G.N. Postma, J.A. Koufman. Validity and reliability of the reflux symptom index (RSI), 274–77, 2002, with permission from Elsevier.

The good news is that this program will help you heal the damage, whether it's severe or just developing, and provide a framework for you to embrace low-acid eating habits for life. And the benefits of the diet are far reaching, extending beyond the immediate acid reflux symptoms and concerns. All of my patients who've tried the Acid Watcher Diet report feeling relief from the pain and disruption of acid damage, increased energy, decreased cravings, and diminished systemic inflammation, which is a precursor of a wide variety of diseases, including type 2 diabetes, hypertension, irritable bowel disease, and rheumatoid arthritis. And, to my great delight, they reported steady and sustainable weight loss.

I was thrilled but not surprised that patients on a low-acid diet lost weight, especially around their midsection, that they otherwise couldn't shed. The Acid Watcher Diet is carefully balanced with healthy macronutrients and a high concentration of fiber. With three meals and two mini-meals, you'll never experience the deprivation that derails so many trying to follow diet plans. Your blood sugar will remain steady, preventing cravings, and your body will be supplied with the optimum amount of vitamins and minerals, such as lycopenes, carotenoids, and flavonoids, helping to accelerate repair of your acid-damaged tissues and cells.

Your action plan to fight back against acid is here, and now it's up to you to put it into use.

PART I

Acid Disruption and Your Diet

CHAPTER 1

Dietary Acid Damage

WHY WE SHOULD ALL FEAR IT

Dietary acid damage is one of the foremost health challenges Americans face, affecting more people than heart disease, diabetes, and celiac disease. Recent statistics reveal that incidence of gastroesophageal reflux disease (GERD), the most common form of acid damage, has more than doubled since 1995; in the United States alone at least sixty million people have acid reflux (the common name for GERD), and worldwide that number leaps to *1.4 billion* people. Some researchers have even gone so far as to declare that a global GERD epidemic is taking place.

Since there are no external signs of acid damage, you may not know how pervasive it is. But experts in gastroenterology and otolaryngology (ear, nose, and throat [ENT]) see it in their patients every day. Even more alarming than the increase in the frequency of the occurrence is the severity of the symptoms. Over the last year, in my practice alone, I have diagnosed Barrett's esophagus, a potentially precancerous condition of the esophageal lining, in nine patients under age thirty. That's a big number for a disease that was once considered rare in people under age fifty, and a startling revelation of how young people with the disease have become. All of these patients had only throat-based symptoms and no heartburn complaints (more on this shortly). Ten years ago this would have been a reportable finding, but not anymore.

Acid Damage 2.0: It's Not Just Heartburn Anymore

What is acid damage? It's a broad range of conditions that contribute to inflammation and disease in various parts of the body. You've likely heard of acid damage in the context of GERD, a condition that a doctor will typically diagnose you with only if you're experiencing the symptoms of heartburn and regurgitation. Surprisingly, though so many people experience the symptoms, they don't always know what causes them. Many of my patients ask: What are heartburn and regurgitation exactly, and how will I feel if I have them?

The simple answer is that *heartburn* occurs when gastric acid from the stomach goes the wrong way, or refluxes, up into the delicate tissues of the esophagus, causing a burning sensation at the bottom of the chest and rib cage that can emanate out through the middle of the chest and toward the throat. *Regurgitation* is the sensation of food coming back up into your chest and throat after you've already swallowed it.

These symptoms are the poster children of acid reflux, but they aren't the only symptoms related to acid damage—in fact, they're not even the most common. In my practice, where we see up to seventy thousand people a month in more than forty different offices, over 90 percent of the people diagnosed with acid reflux disease do not have these typical symptoms. They are more likely to have throat-related complaints such as feeling a lumplike sensation in the throat severe enough to cause dysphagia, or difficulty swallowing. Other common symptoms are chronic cough (which, diagnostically speaking, is cough that persists longer than eight weeks), hoarseness, frequent throat clearing, and sore throat.

If you are experiencing symptoms in which the epicenter of discomfort is your throat, you may have another type of reflux referred to as laryngopharyngeal reflux (LPR), or *throatburn reflux*. The presence of throatburn reflux doesn't mean you're clear of any gastrointestinal acid reflux red flags; in fact, more often than not, a person experiencing throatburn reflux still has heartburn reflux—they just don't know it, because they can't *feel* it. This is because the esophageal tissues have likely been exposed to acid for such a length of time that they've been numbed to its effects. This is a symptom of chronic inflammation (discussed in chapter 3). Only an examination of your esophagus could tell for sure if you have heartburn reflux without knowing it.

Undetected or apparent heartburn reflux, or the nagging throat-centered symptoms, can disrupt your sleep, interfere with your enjoyment of food, annoy your significant other, and affect your energy and activity levels. If, like many of my patients, your voice or public speaking is a source of income, even your livelihood may be affected. What most people don't realize is that their symptoms are the result of years' and sometimes decades' worth of damage that has deteriorated cellular integrity and function, initiated disease-causing chronic inflammation, and, in the most serious cases, created conditions for an aggressive and increasingly common form of cancer of the esophagus. While you may not hear a lot about it now, esophageal cancer will be making news headlines in the years to come—unless we do something to stop it.

The good news is that it's completely within your power to put an end to the symptoms caused by refluxed acid and to curtail the type of internal damage that can leave your esophagus vulnerable to cancer. The solution lies in your diet and learning how to use a different type of measurement than you're accustomed to in order to gauge whether a food or beverage is "good" or "bad" for you. Instead of letting calories, carbohydrates, or fat dictate your dietary choices, the Acid Watcher Diet will teach you to use a substance's acidity or pH value to determine whether it will be harmful or healing to you. This practice, which I call being an Acid Watcher, will help you take back control of your health by alleviating symptoms associated with acid reflux without requiring long-term reliance on over-the-counter or prescription medication.

Whether you realize it or not, you already know a little something about this approach to eliminating symptoms of acid reflux. Have you ever noticed, through trial and error, that certain foods "trigger" your reflux? And that eliminating them has produced some relief, even if it's temporary? Then you've been an Acid Watcher in training all along.

What you probably don't know is that the common understanding of trigger foods doesn't take into account some of the most popular and frequently consumed foods that can cause and worsen acid reflux. You may have been ingesting these foods and beverages every day for months, even years, without knowing that they're contributing to your reflux symptoms. Worse, they could have caused enough damage at this point that your esophagus has been numbed to the effects of refluxed acid—which is why your heartburn symptoms have mysteriously disappeared, while your throat symptoms have flared up.

The substances I'm talking about are processed foods and beverages, and not just any processed foods, but those that have been infused with an invisible chemical known as dietary acid. Many of your favorite items that line the shelves of your grocery store have been acidified, by nature and by chemical process, which means so have you. When dietary acid is added to foods and drinks, the result is a diminished pH value and consequently a greater toxicity to your internal tissues. Most vulnerable to this toxicity is the lining of your esophagus, which is the small tube through which all substances pass before they reach your stomach (you'll learn more about the esophagus in chapter 2).

How Dietary Acid Slipped into Your Every Snack and Meal

Dietary acid is in many of the most commonly consumed foods and drinks, even though you probably don't know it's there. It's in canned and jarred soups and vegetables especially if they've been pickled, marinated, or fermented. It is in all carbonated beverages and industrially produced fruit juices. It's present in every product that contains high-fructose corn syrup, even in items that don't seem to be sweet at all. This ubiquitous and overused sweetener is produced using sulfuric acid and you'll find it in the most unexpected places, such as in condiments, barbecue sauces, cocktail sauces, spice mixes, even baby food.

You'll find dietary acid in breads, salad dressings, juices, yogurts, and candy bars, and in the most deleterious acidic substance of all: soda. And that includes all sugar-free and colorless varieties such as flavored seltzer water, which so many health watchers and dieters falsely presume to be safe.

When you consume, on a daily basis, foods and beverages that contain dietary acid, you invite acid damage into your body. The consequence of letting this seemingly innocuous damage continue eventually turns into more than a postmeal nuisance that a few antacids can control.

Using Food to Heal—and Prevent—Acid Damage

Changing how we eat and what we eat will hasten the healing, recovery, and prevention of acid reflux. The important first step in reversal and prevention of acid damage is to understand where acid originates in our food supply. One general rule to remember is that the more processed the food is, the more severely it is going to exacerbate acid damage to your aerodigestive tract and beyond. (*Aerodigestive* is a medical term for the anatomic pathway from your mouth to your stomach, including your vocal cords, windpipe, and lungs.)

An easy way to gauge the level of processing is to consider how likely you would be to find an item growing on a farm, whether from a tree or plant or in the soil, or in a stream. For example, could you pluck an Oreo as though fruit from a tree, or unearth a bushel of fresh-grown spicy nacho cheese chips? Not in a million years. Will you ever stumble upon a refreshing Coca-Cola-filled creek? Only if you're in a game of Candy Land. It might sound silly, but this thought exercise can be a practical process of elimination when you're selecting what to eat and drink each day.

Of course, an easier way to know what to eat is to follow the eating plan you'll find in this book. The Acid Watcher Diet's primary function is to reduce whole-body acid damage, to help treat acid reflux disease naturally, and to aid in preventing its possible long-term ramifications, including Barrett's esophagus and esophageal cancer. To meet this function, the diet has been designed to be, first and foremost, low-acid. It eliminates a whole range of dangerous processed foods, invites you to expand your table and palate with natural, delicious, and low-acid alternatives, and reins in the destructive sugar cravings.

Yet the fact that it highlights and eliminates high-acid, processed foods from your diet isn't what makes this program a standout in the crowded field of health, diet, and nutrition books. After all, most health-conscious people, whether they are medical professionals or enlightened consumers, already know that processed foods are generally bad for you because, being chemically altered, they are a source of inflammation. There are *three* other angles that give the Acid Watcher program a distinctive edge. First, it identifies food items that are considered healthy by general nutritional standards but are nevertheless extremely harmful to individuals with acid reflux—for example, wine, citrus fruits, raw garlic, raw onion, and tomato. Even the most admired diet plans with a sustained record of benefits—such as the Mediterranean diet—can be bad for Acid Watchers.

The second crucial feature of the Acid Watcher program is that it uses the pH value of foods to identify those that heal or injure consumers in an entirely different way. In other words, just because the food is high in pH doesn't always mean it is good for an Acid Watcher. Read on.

And the third critical feature is that the diet plan is designed to keep pepsin—the enzyme meant to digest food—in your stomach, so that it doesn't wreak havoc on your body if it ends up in the wrong places. If your diet is too acidic—and it is for most people—pepsin is guaranteed to end up in places you don't want it. Pepsin awareness is crucial to fighting dietary acid overload and inflammation.

There are two phases of the Acid Watcher Diet. The first is the Healing Phase, which you will follow for 28 days, the minimum needed to heal the tissue that has been damaged by dietary acid. The second is the Maintenance Phase, in which you can bring back some of the foods that have been excluded from the Healing Phase and set up a solid foundation for an Acid Watcher lifestyle for life. Here's a preview of how each phase will work:

The **Healing Phase** is a 28-day phase that will feature low-acid foods rich in regenerative phytochemicals ideal for repairing damaged esophageal tissue. Guided by the Rule of 5, you will focus on enjoying foods with the pH of 5 and higher, including lean animal proteins, whole grains, and a range of fruits and vegetables; abiding by this principle will help you keep pepsin in check and drastically curtail any continued acid damage. Foods that promote indigestion and acidification will be eliminated, including carbonated beverages, alcohol, caffeine, chocolate, mint, and raw onion and garlic. A variety of delicious, whole foods and low-acid, aromatic herbs and spices will be added to expand your repertoire in the kitchen. With three complete meals and two mini-meals per day, you don't have to worry about feeling hungry or deprived.

Some of my patients initially question the need for 28 days of low-acid eating and have cut short the Healing Phase, especially after they see how quickly it produces desired outcomes of weight loss, higher energy, and bloating reduction. Their improved symptoms trick these patients into thinking that the quick fix has been accomplished. It's important to keep in mind, however, that 28 days is the *minimum* amount of time needed for healing tissues that have been exposed to years, decades, and even a lifetime of acid damage. You will typically begin to feel better early on, with symptoms of indigestion and heartburn and throat clearing beginning to subside in a matter of 21 days (depending on severity), but this is simply evidence that the diet is working, not that it should be over.

Needless to say, those patients who've tried to take a shortcut to success have actually ended up following the Acid Watcher Diet for longer. It takes just one high-acid slipup to slide your progress back. With the detailed 28-day menu guide, the program has been automated for you—make the commitment to yourself to stick with the plan as it is designed.

Two additional benefits are that the menus are meant to be inexpensive (most daily snacks and meals averaging twenty dollars) and preparation time minimal (most recipes are under thirty minutes). Remember: over four thousand patient success stories and counting (and not a one from someone who's cut the diet short). Should you fall off the wagon, rest assured that you were not the first and will not be the last.

The **Maintenance Phase** should last a minimum of two weeks or can be extended for the rest of your life if you want to truly live your best, acid-free life. During this phase, you'll discover strategies for reintroducing caffeine, select alcoholic beverages such as potato- and corn-based vodka, and cooked garlic and onions into the diet. You will get to include slightly more acidic fruits and vegetables and other dietary staples. This includes select dairy products, fruits such as apples and peppers, and sweeteners like honey and the occasional sliver of dark chocolate.

How to Be an Acid Watcher Outside the Kitchen

While swapping damaging, high-acid foods for healing, low-acid ones will be the most important part of your healing process, research and my own clinical experience have proven that a complete recovery from acid damage also includes incorporating lifestyle practices related to exercise, sleep, and stress reduction.

Engaging in exercise that emphasizes stretching, balance, and healing can help neutralize acid damage and promote weight loss—the latter is especially powerful since a 10 percent reduction in weight (if you are overweight or obese) can significantly ease acid-related symptoms.

Research has revealed that poor sleep quality and/or insufficient sleep and chronic stress have a direct relationship to weight gain and acid damage. (You'll learn more about the connection between weight gain and acid reflux in chapter 3.) I'll help you develop awareness about nondietary factors that exacerbate acid damage. For example, how to turn down your body's production of glucocorticoids (GCs), which are a class of steroid hormones released by the body during psychological or emotional stress. When GCs are being produced at a fast clip, the result is greater pepsin production, an increased chance of developing or worsening GERD and stomach ulcers, and a propensity to store more abdominal fat, which is linked to acid reflux and increased chances for developing Barrett's esophagus.

In the chapters to come, you will discover that the Acid Watcher Diet is more than just a food plan (though that is its primary focus); it's a comprehensive lifestyle program that will empower you to heal your body naturally from years of acid damage. The sooner you start the healing, the sooner you will start feeling better.

$$\begin{array}{r} 13\overset{0}{\cancel{3}} \\ -\ 1\,\cancel{3} \\ \hline 1\,1\,7 \end{array}$$

CHAPTER 2

Acid Reflux, Your Esophagus, and the Cancer Connection

The organ that takes the most direct hit from acid damage is the esophagus. Although the damage certainly isn't limited to this important transporter of food and fluids, it's here that the doors to gastric acid can first be left ajar. Gaining a basic understanding of how the esophagus works and its close relationship to the digestive system below it will help you fully grasp the connection between your dietary choices and acid reflux.

You'll also learn about the connection between the rise in acid reflux and the dietary choices that were made *for* you (rather than *by* you) decades ago—the decisions made by food manufacturers in the late 1970s and early 1980s that infused dietary acid into many popular foods and beverages.

Considering the interconnectedness between all of these factors will help put you in the driver's seat of your health.

Meet Your Esophagus—the Organ at the Forefront of Cancer Risk

The esophagus isn't a large organ; in most people, it's only about an inch wide and approximately eight to ten inches in length. Yet this muscular tube could be considered a vital source of life, since it's through this conduit that all nutrients are delivered to your body.

When you eat, chewed food passes through the esophagus and makes its way to the stomach for digestion where it will be further broken down by gastric acid for optimum absorption. Your favorite beverages travel down this path, too, unless of course your voice box or larynx fails to close off the windpipe, or trachea, and a fast-moving guzzle ends up going down the "wrong pipe."

Your esophagus is therefore subject to the effects of what you eat and drink each day before the rest of your body. You might call it a gateway, although it has no screening capabilities or say in the matter on what's allowed: it must let through everything that you eat and drink. The esophagus is lined by pale pink tissue called *mucosa,* which is composed of the same type of epithelial cells that line the inside of your mouth. These are tough cells, meant to withstand abrasion and exposure, but not tough in the way of tooth enamel, the hardest substance in the human body (which, interestingly, can also incur acid damage).

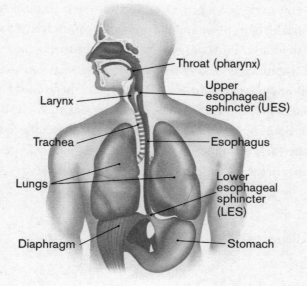

At each end of your esophagus you have a sphincter or muscular shutoff valve. At the upper end you have the upper esophageal sphincter (UES), which is slightly below your Adam's apple, and at the lower end directly above the stomach you have the lower esophageal sphincter (LES), which is approximately where the lower end of your ribs meet.

When we eat or drink, the esophageal sphincters relax and open to allow food and liquids to pass through the throat and down into the stomach. They rely on intricate multidirectional muscle fibers that operate with the intention of creating maximum tension. By design, both the UES and LES are meant to tighten back up once what you've ingested has passed through. In this way, they act as anti-reflux barriers, protecting the tissues above from the corrosive effects of gastric acid.

The epithelial cells lining your esophageal sphincters play a big role in how efficiently and effectively these closures work, specifically in how secure the muscular sphincters are that will work to keep gastric acid in its rightful place: in the stomach below. The esophageal epithelial cells also work together with glands housed in a sublayer of tissue to boost resistance against daily assaults, especially dietary acid exposure. When you ingest highly acidic substances, these glands will secrete neutralizing enzymes to help minimize tissue damage.

Your esophagus has a perfect protective system in place to help preserve the health of its tissue and to ensure that stomach acid doesn't travel where it shouldn't. Problems with reflux begin when the lining of the esophageal sphincters is damaged or eroded by what you consume each day. It's most vulnerable to dietary acid, which I mentioned is the type of acid found in many of today's most popular foods and beverages.

While both the upper and lower sphincters can be affected by regular and repeated acid exposure, they do have varying vulnerabilities. The biggest culprits in the loosening of the LES are the following:

- tobacco
- caffeine
- chocolate
- carbonated sugary drinks
- alcohol

These all contribute to the opening of the door for corrosive gastric acid to reflux from the stomach up into the esophagus. The UES is also susceptible to damage from tobacco and alcohol, and a loss of tension here will allow acid into the upper respiratory organs such as the mouth, larynx, and trachea. Acid in these regions can lead to symptoms that are usually associated with acid reflux, such as the following:

- hoarseness
- phlegm
- postnasal drip
- asthma
- shortness of breath

The Pepsin Problem

Gastric acid, which digests your food in the stomach, rarely travels alone when regurgitated through reflux. When this strong acid flows up into the esophagus and throat, it often brings molecules of pepsin with it, making it even more potent.

Pepsin, an enzyme typically found in the stomach, is triggered to help break down food within the stomach. While acid usually gets most of the attention, even by most medical professionals and pharmaceutical aids (you won't find anti-pepsin medications next to antacids at the drugstore), pepsin presents a very real lurking danger that shouldn't be overlooked.

Pepsin is inactive within the stomach until it's woken up by acidic foods. Once activated and assimilated into gastric acid, it can surge back up into the esophagus, chest, vocal cords, and throat area—made much worse if you have loosened esophageal sphincters. Within the esophagus and throat, the pepsin molecules can attach to pepsin receptors found there, creating a kind of Velcro effect. This is when the real trouble begins.

Once pepsin is planted in your esophagus, it makes itself comfortable and is *activated* each time you eat or drink something acidic. Activated pepsin acts a bit like a hungry Pac-Man and will work quickly to find something to eat or break down. Without the presence of food proteins (which it would normally have to work on in its rightful home, the stomach), pepsin will begin to eat away at the tissues of the throat and esophagus, causing an array of conditions ranging from inflammation and heartburn to Barrett's esophagus, a precancerous condition involving severe acid damage, and possibly esophageal cancer. When pepsin is present, each time you consume highly acidic substances like sugary soda, citrus, or vinegar, *what you eat can literally be eating you.*

The Bad News of Barrett's Esophagus

Barrett's esophagus, or the presence of stomach tissue in the esophagus, is a dangerous sign for patients. It places the individual at a higher risk of developing esophageal cancer. In fact, those with Barrett's esophagus are 30 to 125 times more likely to develop esophageal adenocarcinoma than the general population.

A normal, healthy stomach has an intense pinkish color, like smoked salmon or lox, while the esophageal lining has a grayish-white color. Generally, the pink stomach lining begins where the grayish-white esophagus ends. However, when there is severe acid injury to the bottom portion of the esophagus, the stomach lining starts to creep up into the esophagus, resulting in fingerlike projections of pinkish tissue jutting into the grayish-white esophageal lining.

Barrett's esophagus currently affects roughly 1 percent of adults in the United States. Men typically develop Barrett's esophagus twice as often as women, and it is most common in white males over fifty. However, over the past ten years, I have been seeing men and women in their forties and thirties and even some in their twenties with this condition. Just last year, a twenty-nine-year-old patient referred to me with cough and hoarseness but without heartburn turned out to have Barrett's esophagus.

Eight percent of patients with heartburn reflux (GERD) have Barrett's esophagus. Ominously, up to 10 to 15 percent of throatburn reflux (LPR) patients, those who have no heartburn but do have chronic symptoms of cough, hoarseness, a lumplike sensation in the throat, and throat clearing, have Barrett's esophagus. By "chronic symptoms" I mean symptoms lasting longer than eight weeks.

The Truth About pH

Scientific evidence reveals that the pH value of a substance is what determines the activity level of pepsin, and it's also what determines how damaging a food or drink can be to your esophageal lining. If you remember your high school chemistry class, you may recall that acidity—or the opposite, alkalinity—is measured on the pH scale, which runs from 1 (extremely acidic) to 14 (extremely alkaline). Every substance below pH 7 is considered acidic while everything above pH 7 is considered alkaline. Your body works hard to neutralize the gastric and dietary acid combo to keep the level steady at 7.4.

Research shows that foods and drinks with a pH below 5, and especially those below 4 on the pH scale, will activate pepsin (when we start talking about the diet, you'll discover a list of foods separated by their pH value specifically to help you shut down damaging pepsin activity).

Research links pepsin's presence in the esophageal lining to increased tumor activity, particularly in the area where the lower part of the esophagus joins the stomach.

The Radical Rise of Acid-Related Esophageal Cancer

When I first started practicing medicine, the most common type of esophageal cancer was due to smoking and drinking alcohol. Around the mid-1990s there was a shift in the incidence of esophageal cancer to the type due to acid-mediated injury.

There are two common forms of esophageal cancer—squamous cell carcinoma (SCC) and adenocarcinoma (adenoCA). Both types are often detected late in the malignancy because of a lack of obvious early symptoms. However, there are precancerous changes in the esophagus to watch out for; critically, the Acid Watcher Diet will introduce you to them. In most cases, detection doesn't occur until a patient is experiencing difficulty swallowing because of a developing tumor, which typically forms at an advanced state of the disease. Sadly, the average five-year survival rate at this stage is only 10 to 15 percent.

The two forms of esophageal cancer differ in a number of ways. SCC affects the "flat" cells that line the esophagus and is most likely to arise in the middle to upper regions of the esophagus. AdenoCA affects the glandular cells that release mucus and enzymes to protect the esophageal lining. While adenoCA is also most likely to occur in the middle region of the esophagus, diagnoses of adenoCA in the lower region and in the esophagogastric junction—where the esophagus and the stomach meet—have increased considerably in the last forty years.

This last point is important because it's part of a larger trend and shift in how and why esophageal cancer is manifesting. Before 1970, SCC was the predominant form of esophageal cancer and the cause was relatively clear: 95 percent of patients with squamous cell carcinoma were smokers, and heavy alcohol use was also found to be a contributing factor.

But after 1970, rates of adenoCA began to climb. From the mid-1970s to 1994, incidence of esophageal adenocarcinoma rose 350 percent, and in 1990 it surpassed SCC as the predominant form of esophageal cancer. By 2008, adenoCA had increased an alarming 650 percent, making it the fastest-growing cancer in the United States and Europe.

Smoking wasn't believed to be the cause since it never had as strong a link to adenocarcinoma (and smoking rates were declining during these years), but acid reflux, Barrett's esophagus, and obesity were in the running as contributing factors. Was it possible that dietary factors were behind the startling shift?

What's Behind the Dramatic Increase in Acid Damage?

When we consider the drastic increase in rates of esophageal adenocarcinoma since the 1970s and in rates of other acid-related damage, including acid reflux, throatburn reflux, and Barrett's esophagus, we have to look at what environmental or lifestyle changes were occurring around that time that might have sparked or precipitated the shift from one type of esophageal cancer to another. As it turns out, we don't have to look far at all.

Three food trends in the mid-1970s and early 1980s introduced an unprecedented wave of extremely addictive and unhealthy processed foods, full of not just excess fat, sugar, and calories, but dietary acid, too. These trends helped shape the Western diet as we know it today, and soon after these dietary changes were ushered in, we began to see rates of adenocarcinoma start to surge. Let's explore these trends further.

ACIDIFICATION BY LEGISLATION

In 1975, the Food and Drug Administration (FDA) introduced a law called Title 21, a well-intentioned but ill-thought-out federal legislation that codified and amplified the use of acid in food preservation and prevention of bacterial infection. While we have always relied somewhat on dietary acid to preserve foods safely—think of the use of salts or vinegars to pickle raw goods—Title 21 ensured that acid was infused into far more foods and beverages than ever before. No one predicted or researched thoroughly how this invasion might affect our health in the long term.

According to Title 21 regulations, any raw product with a natural pH of 4.6 or higher (you may recall that this falls right within the pepsin activation window) is considered a "low-acid food" and needs to be immersed in a substance that will transform it into an "acidified" food. Substances used in this preservation process can include acetic acid (vinegar), citric acid, lactic acid, malic acid, phosphoric acid, and in some cases, lye or lime. While the goal is to achieve a shelf-stable pH of 4.6, quite often the finished product will have a pH of 4.2 or lower.

In most cases, you would never know that a food had been acidified. Take, for example, a jar of banana baby food. A banana in its natural form has a pH of around 5.7, while the bananas in a jar are closer to 4. To you, this may not seem like a significant difference. But if you are a scientist or a doctor, you'll know that the pH scale is logarithmic, so the almost two-point difference actually indicates a frightening *hundredfold increase* in acidity. So a child who is eating a jar of baby banana food is consuming a product that is 100 times more acidic than one who is eating a real banana. And this is just at the beginning of life, before the baby's palate will be introduced to an infinite range of processed food and drink. Title 21 made sure that we will ingest acid with our foods from infancy through adulthood—as long as we select glass-bound and canned goods from the grocery-store shelves. And these next food trends extended our acidic exposure even further.

A NEW #1 BEVERAGE IS CROWNED

The same year that acidification became law, soda surpassed coffee as the most popular beverage, a foreboding sign for Acid Watchers everywhere. You've no doubt heard about the health hazards of soda consumption, and the message you've likely received over and over again is that the sugar in soda is the culprit. While this is unequivocally true—sugar is devoid of nutrition and has played a central role in the obesity epidemic—there's another less emphasized villain lurking in soda: acid.

With a pH of around 2.5, soda is the most acidic and corrosive substance we consume—it's so acidic that no living thing would survive in a glass of it overnight. Even if you're not sleeping *in* it, soda will keep you up at night: researchers at the University of Arizona College of Medicine found that consumption of carbonated soft drinks is one of the most common causes of disruptive nighttime heartburn.

When you consume soda, it contributes to acid damage in two ways. First, the intense acidity of the liquid begins to erode your esophageal lining, causing acute damage to the lower esophageal sphincter, which you'll remember has the important job of locking out gastric acid housed in the stomach below. Secondary to the direct acid-caused damage is the effect of carbonation found in sodas. Carbonation amplifies the corrosive quality of soda and works against your acid protection system by increasing pressure in the stomach. As this pressure increases, gastric acid can get refluxed up toward the LES. And since the LES has just been damaged by the downflow of acidic soda, it's essentially been primed to allow for refluxed acid to find its way up onto the tissues of your esophagus. From an Acid Watcher's perspective, soda is enemy number one.

Over the years that soda retained its title as the most popular beverage in the United States, rates of adenocarcinoma skyrocketed. At its peak, soda was being guzzled by the gallons, with the average consumption per person coming in at an astonishing fifty-four gallons per year. Although water knocked soda off the top of the list in 2008, the annual national soda intake is still averaging 44 gallons per year—that's more than is needed to weaken the lower esophageal sphincter and open the door to chronic reflux, Barrett's esophagus, and the cellular dysfunction that can lead to esophageal cancer.

A SUGAR SHIFT OCCURS

If soda was bad for you before 1980, it just got worse from there. That was the year the type of sugar used in processed foods, including soda, went from beet or cane sugar to high-fructose corn syrup (HFCS). What's the problem with HFCS? First of all, it has sulfuric acid in it, which is an extremely acidic substance. Furthermore, the chemicals used in the processing of HFCS have the side effect of loosening the LES.

As the 1980s began, so too did the high-fructose corn syrup invasion. Thanks to corn subsidies, HFCS was far cheaper to produce than other sweeteners and it also proved to be a versatile product, deemed suitable for use in soda, cereal, bread, yogurt, fruit juice, crackers, pickles, salad dressings, barbecue sauces, ketchups, and more. This made it possible for you to get a dose of HFCS—along with some sulfuric acid—not just every day, but in every single meal and snack.

Even just a small amount of sulfuric acid exposure each day could lead to significant esophageal damage over time, paving the way for more serious acid-related issues to develop.

THE CONVENIENCE-FOOD TREND TAKES OFF

Nineteen eighty-three marked the first full year that microwave pop-corn was available to the public. Cooked in bags coated in perfluorooc-tanoic acid (PFOA) and full of other dangerous additives derived from substances like butane, this ready-in-minutes snack epitomized a larger trend toward convenience foods.

This convenience didn't come for free, though. Food manufactur-ers, driven to elevate the flavors of engineered foods and the speed in which they could be made, began to push the chemical envelope even further. An increasing number of food additives and colors were added to processed goods, helping to extend shelf life and, intentionally or not, enhance the addictive quality of a growing number of packaged foods.

Foods such as microwave popcorn, frozen pizzas, and frozen dinners were big hits, and they helped overhaul the way Americans ate. People began to make fewer home-cooked meals and grew to rely heavily on pro-cessed foods, chock-full of artificial ingredients, some now linked to such conditions as attention deficit/hyperactivity disorder (ADHD), asthma, and headaches. The use of additives and preservatives accelerated from the 1980s on—you'll now find over three thousand items listed in the FDA's database of food additives, synthetic flavors, and colors.

Assessing the Damage and Exploring Opportunities for Change

Over the decades since these food trends were introduced, rates of weight gain have climbed significantly. It's no surprise, since eating processed foods doesn't just come with greater acid exposure and ingestion of food additives, it's also a guaranteed way to consume excess sugar, saturated fat, trans fats, and calories, making weight gain all but inevitable. And this weight gain in turn has contributed to a type of metabolic dysfunc-tion that has links first to high blood pressure, insulin resistance, and high cholesterol, and later to chronic diseases such as cardiovascular dis-ease and type 2 diabetes.

In the next chapter, I'll explore the relationship between dietary acid and a constellation of these medical conditions, and what could be the perilous problem linking them together: chronic inflammation. The Acid Watcher Diet is about keeping your dietary acid *and* your inflammation low. Poor dietary choices and inflammation always go hand in hand. Even if you don't have a severe form of acid damage (such as a precancerous condition like Barrett's esophagus), if you partake of the processed-food-rich standard American diet, you are most likely experiencing some form of inflammation. This diet will help you relieve it.

Keep reading to discover what you need to know about inflammation and how diet plays into the equation—as a problem (dietary acid), and as a solution (low-acid, antioxidant-rich foods).

CHAPTER 3

Inflamed

THE LINKS BETWEEN INFLAMMATION, ACID REFLUX, AND WEIGHT GAIN

Patients who come to see me have already experienced the classic symptoms of acid reflux disease—sometimes for years—in their larynx where the vocal cords live, their throat, and esophagus. They describe symptoms like a persistent cough, hoarseness, feeling an obstruction or lump in their throat, or heartburn. When I ask questions about their overall health they tell me about additional problems—fatigue, joint pain, and high blood pressure, to name a few. On the surface these additional ailments do not seem to be linked to their acid reflux. So when I tell my patients that the Acid Watcher Diet may, in addition to healing direct acid-induced injuries, help relieve other symptoms as well, they seem surprised.

But it does happen. I remember one patient in particular, a fifty-two-year-old social worker named Leanne who came to me in hopes of finding a cure for a lumplike sensation in her throat that had bothered her for the previous two years. Leanne also reported experiencing heartburn, bloating, and irritable bowel syndrome (IBS). She had been recently diagnosed with celiac disease, but a strict gluten-free diet did not improve her symptoms significantly. And lastly, Leanne mentioned having psoriasis, an autoimmune disease that produces scaly, uncomfortable, and sometimes painful red blotches on the skin.

I suspected that Leanne's digestive problems continued because, even though she had gone gluten free, she still continued to consume caffeinated products, chocolate, raw onion, garlic, tomatoes, and wine. Some of her daily routines weren't exactly helpful to relieving heartburn. For example, like most working people with multiple responsibilities, Leanne ate dinner late in the evening, at about 9:00 p.m., approximately two hours before going to bed. Gluten free or not, eating so close to bedtime was going to produce some flowback of food and gastric juices back into the esophagus, as the stomach takes about three to four hours to empty.

Because Leanne had symptoms of throatburn and heartburn, I put her on the Acid Watcher Diet, excluding a handful of items that contain gluten. After three months on the diet Leanne came back to my office for a follow-up. Predictably, the lumplike sensation in her throat had dissolved. She had lost weight—nine pounds and a half inch from her waist—and found relief from heartburn, bloating, and IBS symptoms. But the change that stood out the most was not the relief from acid reflux injuries that I predicted; it was Leanne's aside that her psoriasis was improving as well. Even more startling was the revelation that Leanne's older sister, who also had psoriasis (but not heartburn), joined her on the Acid Watcher Diet. And her psoriasis symptoms improved as well!

Naturally, I asked myself how a diet designed to heal acid reflux injury could also help relieve symptoms of an autoimmune disease like psoriasis. This brought up a bigger question: What does acid damage have to do with other dysfunctions throughout the body? The physiological mechanisms in the body are densely intertwined. Dietary acid doesn't just affect the organs and systems immediately in its path; it can also reflect, trigger, and illuminate other disruptions that unfold multilaterally in the body at all times. The trick is to find the root cause for why and how the disruption happens.

The root cause of most disruptions in the body is inflammation. To grasp the extent of how dietary acid can both create and exacerbate inflammation, you have to know a few basics about how your body works. While this book isn't meant to be a biology or organic chemistry primer, stick with me through these pages and you will better understand the connection between some of your medical problems and dietary acid injury. More importantly, you will better understand the rationale behind the Acid Watcher program and see why sticking to it will help you manage and prevent health and medical challenges beyond throatburn and heartburn—that is, *beyond acid reflux disease.*

Inflammation 101

Inflammation is your body's complicated response to physiological stress, toxic exposure, or trauma. Think of it as a state of agitation ranging anywhere from mild to extreme, from completely imperceptible to the kind that leaves you howling in pain.

Over the last century, inflammation has become the holy grail of medicine and science as it can affect all of our anatomical systems and is believed to be ground zero for a wide range of medical conditions and diseases. If there is a code to how inflammation translates into disease, then unlocking it will undoubtedly revolutionize how we prevent and cure disease. For now, we only know one thing for sure: inflammation is a precursor to a range of autoimmune, metabolic, and chronic diseases. Dietary acid injury clearly illuminates this connection.

Before we go any further it is important to distinguish between two kinds of inflammation—**acute inflammation,** which can be helpful, and **chronic inflammation,** which is not. One example of acute inflammation is when your sprained ankle swells up and puts you on the sidelines for at least a few days. That swelling is a sign that an inflammatory response has been cued: white blood cells and hormones have been rushed to the injured area to clear out any infection or tissue damage and to begin the healing process. In this case, the inflammation serves as a warning to be careful with a body part undergoing trauma and as a healing mechanism. When the healing process is complete, the swelling will subside and the ankle will be back to normal.

Chronic inflammation is a more insidious condition because, unlike acute inflammation, it isn't temporary nor is it obvious. This type of inflammation often occurs in response to low-grade, persistent exposure to toxins such as pesticides, dietary acid, and cigarette smoke, or to an unresolved infection. Chronic inflammation can be severe and progressive, as the body perceives that a nearly constant threat is present. In this case, your white blood cells, which are designed to remove damaged tissue and then clear out, instead loiter around. They then robotically try and clear out injured tissue, often taking out nearby healthy tissue as collateral damage. The process is destructive, and sadly it announces itself—if it announces itself at all—only when it is in full swing.

Scarier still is that you never know where chronic inflammation will strike. It can chew up the nerve cells in your brain (Alzheimer's disease), direct the depositing of cholesterol into your coronary arteries (heart attack), make you insulin resistant (type 2 diabetes), or make you hack from acid injury to your vocal cords (throatburn).

The question is: What's the spark that sets the eternal flame of chronic inflammation ablaze? It all begins with the birth of free radicals.

The Birth of Free Radicals, Your Body's Rogue Cells

When the body is exposed to such things as air pollution, ultraviolet rays, and toxins like dietary acid and cigarette smoke, it reacts first and foremost on a cellular level. The trauma from such exposure can cause molecules to lose single electrons, giving birth to a highly reactive and unstable by-product called a free radical. These free radicals crave stability and immediately seek out a replacement electron, bumping into and hoping to bond with the first free-floating molecules with which they come into contact. In many cases, the first free molecule encountered will be oxygen-based, resulting in an altered, oxidized molecule that doesn't function quite like it used to.

There is growing evidence that free radicals—which are also the agents of aging—are implicated in cellular injury throughout the body, damaging whatever tissue they target. They are also capable of disrupting DNA and creating a gene mutation that may eventually transform a normal cell into a malignant one. Their presence has been linked to the development of common ailments, including cardiovascular diseases, neurodegenerative diseases, metabolic syndrome, and cancer.

Let's take a brief look at how the process unfolds.

The Oxidizing Effect

Oxygen is one of the most abundant elements in the universe and is essential to the life of all aerobic species. So you might wonder how the process of oxidation that occurs as free radicals are formed can be a bad thing. The simplest way to understand it is to think about the chemical process of browning that occurs in fruits and vegetables that have been exposed to air. A whole pristine apple can sit in a nonrefrigerated fruit bowl for two to four weeks before showing signs of deterioration. Yet as soon as you cut the apple, the cells that have been damaged by your knife will seek out and bond to free-floating oxygen molecules, thus activating the browning or deteriorating process. Similarly, when stressors such as dietary acid, cigarette smoking, pollution exposure, and disease-causing pathogens damage the cells inside our bodies, the injured cells become reactive and vulnerable to oxidation. Oxidized cells "brown" in their own way, losing strength, quality, and sense of function, and begin to accelerate or exacerbate the deterioration of tissues.

Although we can't control the process entirely, we can help our bodies fight oxidation through a diet rich in phytochemicals (found in fruit and vegetable plants), which are natural antioxidants. Vitamins A, C, and E and minerals like copper, zinc, and selenium have been known to help, though less so than a long-term, healthy diet.

The Progression to Reactive Oxygen Species (ROS) and Oxidative Stress

Molecules altered by free radicals are referred to as reactive oxygen species (ROS). ROS will naturally look to donate oxygen to other substances, promoting oxidation, which is a sort of "browning" or aging. In the body, this cellular aging is counterbalanced by **antioxidants,** which are enzymes our body produces on its own or takes in through food and supplements. A balance between oxidants and antioxidants is essential for optimum health, and trouble begins when the scales tip in favor of free radicals. In this environment, where the "bad guys" (ROS) outnumber the good (antioxidants), a state of **oxidative stress** sets in. With oxidative stress comes a dangerous imbalance that can adversely affect individual organs and biological processes in the body.

What You Need to Know About Antioxidants

There are two types of antioxidants: enzymatic (already present in your body) and nonenzymatic, which you can consume in the form of nutritional supplements and food. Some of the more common nonenzymatic supplements are vitamins A, C, and E; beta-carotene; and minerals such as zinc, copper, and selenium.

- Vitamin C has been associated with reduced cardiovascular disease and lower cholesterol, as it interferes in the low-density lipoprotein (LDL) oxidation process. LDL carries cholesterol in the blood. It is also known as "bad cholesterol" because elevated amounts lead to plaque build-up in arteries thereby contributing to stroke and heart attack.

- Vitamin E has also been shown to increase LDL oxidative resistance.

- Flavonoids—found in most fruits, vegetables, dried beans, teas, and grains—also fight oxidation. They have been shown to play a protective role in improving neuronal activity and treatment of diabetes.

Research shows that long-term consumption of dietary antioxidants as opposed to sporadic boosts provided by vitamins and supplements can lower the effects of oxidative DNA damage throughout, decreasing your overall chances of inflammation and susceptibility to viruses, allergies, and cancer. That is why I recommend diet over supplements in treating acid damage and reducing whole-body inflammation.

The Immune System Response

Because oxidative stress happens on the molecular level, we aren't aware of the internal trouble. Our immune system, however, is, and it pulls the trigger on an inflammatory response to the threat of persistent low-grade oxidative stress.

You'll remember that in the best-case scenario an army of problem-clearing white blood cells will get called out to address a threat, do their job, and then retire. But in the case of oxidative stress, free-radical-altered cells can set off false alarms and draw immune cells out to a location where they're not really needed. In this case, warrior white cells will inflame tissues without resolving the problem; worse, they are creating problems as they battle against an imagined enemy. This is the origin of autoimmune disease.

The immune system itself is not immune to subversion; it may become a target of radicalization by the rogue cells, generating even more free radicals as it goes into battle. With this kind of programming and reprogramming capability, free radicals, inflammation, and immune system dysfunction can form a dangerous alliance.

Inflammation and Malignancy Link

When oxidative stress is no longer low grade, things can go from bad to worse, especially when the sustained cellular damage leads to the first molecular sparks of cancer. There is convincing evidence that free radicals can play a role in all stages of cancer development, from initiation, to promotion, to progression. Free radicals can cause mutations in crucial genes (initiation), stimulate cell division (promotion), and in the later stages of carcinogenesis (progression) enable the accumulation of additional DNA damage that can transition a benign cell into a malignant one. Because of this far-reaching level of involvement, there is little doubt in the medical community that oxidative stress is a base from which cancerous growth spurs.

The Dietary Acid Factor in Whole-Body Inflammation

At this point, you're likely wondering what dietary acid has to do with inflammation and all its consequences. Interestingly, acid reflux disease is an especially good example of how dietary acid, oxidative stress, and inflammation interact and develop because they do so on acute and chronic levels.

Let's look at dietary acid in the **acute inflammation** scenario: When you regularly consume high-fructose corn syrup, sweetened carbonated drinks, or canned, processed food filled with preservatives, you are introducing pathogens into your body that create free radicals and eventually oxidative stress. The resulting injury can result in the inflammation of your vocal cords, for one. The vocal cords will swell up in response to repeat infusion of acidic drinks, and this acute inflammation will make you hoarse. If you smoke, this acute inflammation can be made even worse.

Heartburn is also an example of acute inflammation in the digestive tract. The burning you feel in your chest is the inflammatory response to gastric acid injuring the esophagus. In the morning, coffee regurgitating into the esophagus could bring on the burn. At night, it could be the dinner you enjoyed too late into the evening creeping up, along with the gastric juices from the stomach into your esophagus as you are trying to fall asleep.

Another example of acid-induced acute inflammation can occur in the respiratory tract when the acid refluxing from the stomach literally spills into the tissue of the lung, causing *aspiration*. I'll discuss aspiration in greater detail in chapter 4, but suffice it to say that the symptoms—choking, obstruction-of-breath sensations—are very unpleasant.

An unmistakable sign of acid-reflux-induced **chronic inflammation** is the presence of dietary acid molecules in organs where they clearly do not belong—for example, in the lung. How does acid travel from the esophagus in your digestive tract to the lung, which is in your respiratory tract? This happens when pepsin that's been activated in the stomach ends up in the esophagus, and from there it starts to float. And when pepsin floats, it can end up anywhere, including in the lungs, where it can initiate lung inflammation and conditions such as asthma and bronchitis.

For an Acid Watcher, it is especially important to understand that pepsin is not just damaging to the esophagus. It can end up in other tissues as well, bringing acid-induced inflammation along with it. Repeatedly exposing your body to a high volume of dietary acid will inevitably lead to pepsin activation and help create the conditions for whole-body inflammation. And, if you are experiencing other health problems, acid reflux will make them even more challenging.

Acid Reflux, Obesity, and Metabolic Disruption

One of the long-term side effects of the Title 21 legislation that its architects couldn't have anticipated back in the 1970s was the metabolic disruption that would result from the ingestion of the acidified, chemically altered, processed products in our food supply. Some of the medical crises we are currently facing as a nation—and increasingly, globally—are the trifecta of obesity, GERD, and metabolic syndrome and their attendant disorders: type 2 diabetes and cardiovascular disease. Each of the three can reinforce the others, and all share the following features in common: dietary acid and inflammation.

Consider obesity. As a medical condition, obesity is characterized as an increase in body weight that results in excessive fat accumulation, with a body mass index (BMI) of 30 or higher. Obesity, once established, also becomes a destructive catalyst for other dysfunction.

You don't have to be a medical professional to observe the increase in the rates of obesity, but the statistical evidence is there. According to Nutrition Science Initiative, a nonprofit organization dedicated to the study of obesity and type 2 diabetes, the rate of obesity in the United States increased 200 percent between 1970 and 2011. This time line also reflects the transitional period in the nutritional landscape of the United States, which occurred since the passage of Title 21.

Calculating Your BMI

It is always a good idea to get your BMI measured during your annual physical exam, but if you can't wait a second longer, you can go to the following website, which will perform the calculation for you. See http://www.cdc.gov/healthyweight/assessing/bmi/adult_bmi/english_bmi_calculator/bmi_calculator.html.

One dangerous feature of being overweight, if not outright obese, is the accumulation of fat around the belly, otherwise known as visceral fat. Abdominal obesity, defined as a waistline of more than about thirty-four inches, is often supported by visceral fat cells that are now known to be hormonally and metabolically disruptive.

Visceral fat cells can produce free radicals that secrete faulty messenger proteins (hormones), which command your body to store fat rather than convert it to energy. Then, to add insult to injury, they send a message to your brain that you are still hungry even when your belly is as full as it can be. This creates a vicious cycle: The more visceral fat you have, the hungrier you feel because the hormones are sending the wrong message to your brain. The more you eat, the more food you ingest. The more food you ingest, the greater portion will be stored as fat. The more fat you store, the heavier you become. Especially in the abdominal region.

Obesity, GERD, and Esophageal Cancer Links

As an Acid Watcher, you need to pay attention to weight gain, especially in the abdominal region, because of its connection to the development of gastroesophageal reflux disease (GERD). Research published in the *New England Journal of Medicine* has shown that as BMI rises, so does the risk for developing GERD. A person with a BMI in the overweight range was found to be almost twice as likely to have GERD compared with a normal-weight individual. Obese individuals, those with a BMI of 30 or higher, had nearly triple the risk of experiencing gastroesophageal reflux.

GERD, like obesity, is a growing epidemic. Studies show that close to 20 percent of adults in the Western world exhibit GERD symptoms. And there are indications that unless something changes, it will climb higher. A 2007 meta-analysis of reports published over the past twenty years revealed that the prevalence of GERD has increased by 4 percent per year globally, and in North America, the incidence increased 5 percent annually between 1992 and 2005. This means that on average, over the last quarter century or so, the U.S. population has experienced an increase in acid reflux incidence faster and in greater numbers than the rest of the world. And, lest we forget, the rates of obesity over the same period have soared as well.

These statistics don't surprise me, given our reliance on fast and processed foods that are high in acid, fat, and calories. But the questions remain: How can being obese predispose one to GERD (or vice versa)? Or, how can being obese exacerbate the existing symptoms of GERD?

The simplest explanation is that accumulating fat, especially in the abdominal region right beneath the lower esophageal sphincter (LES), interferes with the muscle's function of keeping the acid in the stomach and out of the esophagus. To visualize this scenario, imagine putting pressure on a water-filled balloon around its opening. Doing so will force some of the water up and out of the balloon. The same thing happens around the junction between your stomach and esophagus. When fat accumulates beneath the LES, the contents of the stomach backflow from the stomach into the esophagus, creating acid reflux. If you are inactive— let's say lying down after a meal—the force of gravity kicks in, making the effect even more certain.

We know that repeated acid injury to the esophagus that comes from GERD can lead to Barrett's esophagus, a precancerous condition. A recent study by the American College of Gastroenterology confirms that GERD is a risk factor for the development of Barrett's esophagus. And being obese, especially morbidly obese, defined by a BMI of 35 or higher, places one at even higher risk of developing GERD as well as precancerous and cancerous conditions of the esophagus. A study conducted by researchers with the Baylor College of Medicine determined that obesity *more than doubled* the risk for developing esophageal adenocarcinoma.

With incidence rates for all three conditions—obesity, GERD, and esophageal cancer—increasing, isolating a cause and finding a cure has become a major public health priority. What we know so far is that inflammation is one feature they share.

The Urgency of Dietary Solutions for Fighting Whole-Body Inflammation

Decoding the relationship between oxidative stress, inflammation, and diseases such as autoimmune dysfunction, metabolic disruption, obesity, GERD, and cancer is still a work in progress. We don't have a magic bullet, but we know there are preventive measures we can take to help reduce exposure to oxidative stress, thereby decreasing our chances of chronic inflammation and its attendant complications. And we know that *food is the medicine* that can relieve some of the effects of inflammation.

The Acid Watcher Diet is naturally anti-inflammatory in its immediate and long-term effects. In the short term, the elimination of dietary acid—found in some natural products and all processed foods—will help you reduce and heal pepsin-induced inflammation that causes potentially painful tissue damage in the larynx, throat, and esophagus. And in the long term, adhering to this high-antioxidant, low-acid diet will fight the disease-causing free radicals throughout your body, reducing the risk of chronic inflammation and disease. And lastly, the Acid Watcher Diet is high in fiber, so it will keep you satiated, help you lose extra pounds, and keep the scourge of obesity at bay.

It is never too late to start reducing inflammation throughout your body. And you never know the extent of the benefits you'll experience until you spend the 28 days on my program. Just as Leanne—the patient I wrote about at the start of the chapter—discovered that the Acid Watcher Diet relieved her psoriasis symptoms, you may find relief from some of your inflammation-related discomforts. In Leanne's case—and in the case of her sister—it was psoriasis. In your case, it may be another problem, such as rheumatoid arthritis or Crohn's disease (autoimmune disorders), weight gain (a metabolic disruption), or high blood pressure (cardiovascular disease). Fighting inflammation is always a positive step to take. And doing this through diet and habit adjustment will benefit you in ways you can't even foresee.

As I've already said, I believe that a dietary solution is the most direct and reliable path to preventing and healing acid damage. If, however, acid damage is advanced, a medical evaluation and medicinal treatment are critical and must be done correctly in order to be effective. In the next chapter I will provide an overview of the available diagnostic and medical prescriptions available for people with acid reflux. I will also outline the challenges the medical community—and patients—are facing in successfully treating acid-related disease.

CHAPTER 4

Seeking Treatment

WHAT YOU SHOULD KNOW WHEN YOU SEE
YOUR DOCTOR WITH A THROAT COMPLAINT

I f you've had symptoms of acid reflux for some time, you're familiar with the frustration that comes with the condition. In addition to the physical discomfort you are experiencing, there is the sinking feeling that you may never again know what it's like to be unburdened by your symptoms. And the worst part is, this feeling remains even after you've already been to a few doctors. Unfortunately, I see patients just like you every day.

Currently, there are fundamental challenges in identifying and treating the many manifestations of acid damage. The predominant problem, which I mentioned earlier, is the narrow understanding of what symptoms indicate possible acid damage. In many cases, doctors misunderstand the red-flag symptom of chronic cough—that is, a cough that has been going on for eight weeks—or they overlook other throat-centered signs of acid damage because no heartburn is present. Yet, as you know by now, symptoms outside the gastrointestinal region can indicate a more advanced form of acid reflux.

Because of the confounding nature of the disease, missed diagnoses and incorrect diagnoses occur with alarming frequency, and treatment is often either incorrect or poorly adhered to—typically because patients don't understand the severity of their symptoms, or the risks of letting them continue on unchecked. (If you've been following along up until this point in the Acid Watcher Diet, you are already far ahead of these patients and most of the people who land in my office as you understand the precancerous potential of acid damage.)

If you are seeking medical evaluation and treatment, the following information should help you avoid the pitfalls of those who have gone before you and gain a deeper understanding of how symptoms of acid damage manifest. You'll also discover when to see a doctor and what your options are in the diagnostic process.

Let's start by taking a look at the common and frustrating path far too many patients land on when seeking solutions to atypical reflux symptoms. If it looks familiar to you, don't worry; you're now on the right track to feeling better.

The Throatburn Reflux (Not-So) Merry-Go-Round

Both patients and primary care doctors overlook gastric acid as the cause of throatburn. More often than not, symptoms that are present in the upper aerodigestive tract—the lungs, throat, and head—can land a person with reflux on the throatburn reflux merry-go-round. It usually looks a bit like this:

1. First, the patient attributes cough, hoarseness, or hacking, or in some cases shortness of breath, to other causes like asthma, allergies, colds, or bronchial infection, and seeks treatment from a general practitioner. Remember that mucus or nasal drip can be a symptom of something else coming up from the body.

2. Second, a general practitioner may not detect the stomach connection in what seems like a pulmonary set of symptoms and, as a consequence, directs a patient to the incorrect specialist.

3. Third, specialists tend to focus on the part of the body within their professional expertise; if, for example, a pulmonary specialist doesn't see a problem in the upper chest or throat, he or she

may erroneously clear the patient. In the meantime, the damage will only get worse.

If you've landed on this not-so-merry-go-round (or know someone who has), you know it is relentless, costly, and time consuming. It can also begin to erode your trust in physicians. Yet these inconveniences pale in comparison to the greater risk of delayed treatment: the unregulated continuance of the precancerous condition of Barrett's esophagus. Research now shows that patients who have experienced ten or more years of throatburn symptoms but have few to no GERD symptoms are at increased risk for developing both Barrett's esophagus and esophageal adenocarcinoma. Two other groups at particular risk are those who have had ten or more years of mild GERD symptoms who have not been medically treated and those with ten or more years of mild GERD symptoms who have been medically treated with proton pump inhibitors (PPIs), drugs designed to reduce gastric acid production. Patients who present this potential *trifecta of trouble*—(1) atypical symptoms and/or (2) mild typical GERD symptoms without treatment and/or (3) mild typical GERD symptoms with treatment—are more likely to have the type of severe acid damage that can lead to the development of esophageal cancer.

If I had to select one message from this book to shout from the rooftops, this would be it—if we are ever going to gain ground on the fastest-growing cancer in the world, throatburn symptoms must be connected with acid damage, not just in physicians' minds but in patients' as well. Let's take a closer look at the many ways acid damage can manifest in the throat and in the broader region of the aerodigestive tract.

The Complete List of Throatburn Reflux Symptoms (and How They Happen)

If you've heard of throatburn reflux at all, it's likely under the name of *silent reflux*, which is a glaring example of mislabeling. Not only are many of the symptoms of throatburn reflux quite audible, especially those of coughing, hacking, and throat clearing, but *silent* also suggests a sort of invisibility, which is a dangerous way to characterize a condition that has been linked to cancer.

The clinical name of throatburn reflux is laryngopharyngeal reflux (LPR), so called because symptoms are most often experienced when acid from the stomach is refluxed into the region where the larynx and pharynx meet. The larynx, also known as the voice box, houses the vocal cords and plays an important role in respiration by letting air pass through while keeping foods and beverages out of the vital airway. The pharynx, commonly known as the throat, includes three sections: the top or nasopharynx, which connects to the nasal cavity; the middle or oropharynx, which is adjacent to the mouth; and the bottom or laryngopharynx, which opens to the larynx and esophagus. LPR refers more specifically to this bottom section, but since these are relatively close quarters (see the figure below), acid can easily expand its reach into the mouth, sinuses, middle ear, and lungs (via the trachea), where it can exacerbate conditions such as asthma and recurrent pneumonia.

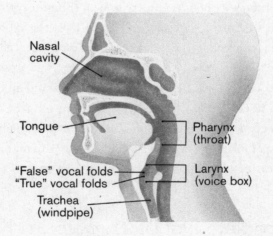

Throatburn reflux symptoms occur when both the lower and upper esophageal sphincters have weakened to the point that they let gastric acid pass beyond the esophagus and farther up into places it doesn't belong. The throat is extremely sensitive to acid exposure. Even a single episode of acid hitting the throat can transform the vulnerable tissues found here. When acid reaches the vocal folds (aka vocal cords), these normally thin and delicate membranes, which vibrate to help produce sound when you speak or sing and close off when needed to protect the lungs, gradually turn into thick, swollen, sausagelike structures. This swelling and irritation may lead to coughing and hoarseness and create other issues in the throat, such as mucus buildup, which can contribute to a lumplike sensation, trouble swallowing, and frequent throat clearing. Here is a full list of symptoms that have been linked to throatburn reflux:

Throatburn Reflux Symptoms

- Hoarseness
- Frequent throat clearing
- Acidic taste in the mouth: acid regurgitation from the stomach can literally bring an acidic taste all the way into the mouth
- Globus sensation: feeling a lump in the throat or that something is stuck in the throat
- Trouble swallowing
- Chronic cough
- Aspiration: food or saliva or any other material going into lungs
- Waking up at night due to burning in the throat
- Waking up at night with a choking sensation
- Excessive mucus in the throat

If you experience any of the preceding symptoms for longer than two weeks, you should see a doctor. The only exception to this rule is chronic cough. See "The Complicated Matter of Chronic Cough" later in this chapter for more information on this frustrating symptom.

A critical reminder: heartburn and regurgitation are not the only symptoms of acid in your esophagus. If you don't feel the effects of acid in your esophagus, this does not mean the discomfort in your throat is not caused by acid. What it means instead is that your esophagus has likely been numbed so severely by repeated acid exposure that you are frighteningly unaware of the ongoing damage taking place. For this reason, persistent throat-related symptoms should be considered the true alarm symptoms of dangerous damage in the esophagus.

Acid damage can extend into your windpipe or worse, your lungs, if the amount of gastric acid is considerable. When the protective reflex

What Your Doctor May See: Acid Damage at a Glance

When you experience damage to any external tissue, it's easy to see—cuts and scrapes become red, bloody, even swollen, and possibly later develop into pus or bruising. You know that something has happened because you can see the evidence with your own eyes, and you feel compelled to care for the injury partly because of this visible proof. When you experience damage to internal tissue, the motivation to take healing action is diminished at least somewhat by the proverbial problem of "out of sight, out of mind."

Patients who hear that their larynx is swollen often ask what "normal" tissue looks like compared to swollen. I usually use images or drawings such as these to demonstrate the difference, and they can be a powerful motivator to start and stick with the diet. Here, you too can see the difference between a normal larynx and an acid-injured larynx.

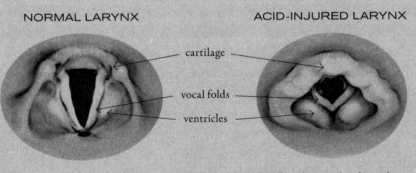

NORMAL LARYNX   ACID-INJURED LARYNX

cartilage

vocal folds

ventricles

In the normal larynx, one can easily identify the entire length of both the right and left vocal folds which come together in a

V-shape at the front of the larynx. The vocal folds are thin, white structures like a violin or banjo string with a black line on each side of them. The black line represents an air space between the true vocal folds and the overlying false vocal folds, called the ventricles.

In the acid-injured larynx, one can only see the front half of the true vocal folds. The back half is "hiding" underneath swollen cartilage. The true vocal folds themselves are also swollen like kielbasa or sausages. The space between the true and false vocal folds is obliterated because the vocal folds are now very inflamed, and the entire structure has become puffy and ill defined. The acid-damaged tissue has become so swollen that it hangs over the trachea or airway, narrowing the actual airway by almost half, which can affect consumption of food and beverages and respiration.

of the vocal folds is overwhelmed by a significant sloshing of acid, the interloping substance can get splashed into the lungs, causing a choking sensation. The entrance of any substance other than air into the lungs is called *aspiration*. All too often, this acid-lung exposure occurs in the middle of the night while you're sleeping (because the supine position can leave you more vulnerable to refluxed acid). You've had this experience if you've ever woken up in a sudden choking panic, gasping for air. My patients refer to these nocturnal choking episodes as "jump-ups" because the experience leaves them jumping up out of bed desperate to regain their breath.

If acid continues to spill into the lungs for an ongoing period of time, it can lead to compromised respiration and complicate issues with asthma, pneumonia, and other lung diseases. The problem worsens when pepsin molecules travel into the respiratory region as well. This "floating" pepsin can settle into bronchial tissues and deepen the damage, setting the stage for chronic inflammation in the lungs.

One common throatburn reflux symptom that is frequently misinterpreted as a lung-related symptom is chronic cough. While chronic

My Own Startling Experience with Reflux

One night in the fall of 1996, I was suddenly awakened by the sensation of someone choking me. I couldn't breathe. The more I tried to inhale, the less air I could take in. I immediately started to panic. I was in my midthirties and about to be married, with hopes of having children one day. As I gasped for air, my mind raced with fear. Was this how I was going to die—suddenly, in the middle of the night, with my fiancée sleeping peacefully beside me? What was going on?

I knew that I had only a few moments before I was going to pass out from a lack of oxygen to my brain. I had to do something. Instinctively, I compressed my lips tightly and started to slowly inhale through my nose, taking steady deep breaths. This gave me the oxygen that my body craved. Thankfully, this steady closed-lip sniff relaxed the spasm in my throat and the choking stopped.

So what had happened to me? At the time, I was the director of the Division of Head and Neck Surgery at the Columbia Presbyterian Medical Center in New York. I was an ear, nose, and throat (ENT) physician and surgeon who specialized in swallowing disorders, as well as in performing surgery to excise cancers of the head and neck. How could I, an expert in diagnosing and treating throat and breathing problems, have nearly suffocated in my own bed without a single warning sign?

I soon learned the startling reason for my choking episode. It was due to a form of acid reflux disease that rarely presents itself with traditional symptoms such as heartburn and regurgitation. *How could I have had acid reflux but no heartburn?* Even my personal physician wouldn't accept this as a possibility. "It's got to be something else. After all, you've never even complained about having heartburn!"

Unfortunately, he was wrong. But luckily, my disease turned out to be reversible at the stage at which it was diagnosed. This frightening experience started me on a path to recognize the otherwise overlooked and almost invisible symptoms of acid reflux disease in patients who were attending my own clinical practice in New York.

Since then, I have seen and treated thousands of patients with acid reflux disease who, like me, didn't experience heartburn or regurgitation. My personal journey with acid reflux disease started first with an awareness of what was happening to me, and at first I used medications to treat my symptoms. Over the years I used a trial-and-error method to stay away from foods and lifestyles (e.g., eating late) that seemed to trigger symptoms. But it wasn't until several years after my initial event that I began to use diet as the bedrock of how to manage this disease.

cough can result from upper-respiratory-tract infection or chronic airway inflammation otherwise known as chronic bronchitis, it can also occur when the throat is continually exposed to acid. Perilously, most people, including far too many doctors, don't associate chronic cough with acid reflux. But as Bill's story shows us, making this connection could save lives.

The Complicated Matter of Chronic Cough

Bill is a sixty-two-year-old advertising executive who is a lifetime non-smoker. Beginning at age fifty, he did his best to pay attention to his health. He made sure to get a routine screening colonoscopy every five years, and each year he had an annual visit to his primary physician as well. The one problem he had was a chronic cough, which he'd been dealing with for ten years. He had two chest X-rays that were negative. He had tried treating it with over-the-counter antihistamines, decongestants, and cough medicine, but nothing seemed to help. It wasn't until his most recent routine colonoscopy when a nurse at the facility asked him how long he'd been coughing. "Ten years," Bill said. The nurse suggested that they get approval from his gastroenterologist to perform an upper endoscopy as well. Since Bill had wanted to get to the bottom of his cough for years, he agreed to the nurse's plan.

A week later, the results of the two tests came back: his colonoscopy was negative for any abnormalities, but the upper endoscopy revealed esophageal cancer with lymph node metastasis.

As a medical professional, I look at Bill's esophageal cancer diagnosis and I see the cracks in the system. If only his gastroenterologist had asked about his throat symptoms or his primary care doctor had gotten a little more inquisitive about the chronic cough. (Then again, when you have a cough the last thing a patient thinks about is discussing it with their gastrointestinal doctor.) Further, with negative chest X-rays the chronic cough might seem harmless or an environmental-related nuisance. While it may be tempting to try to suppress a cough (or postpone a doctor's visit) with cough drops, lozenges, and syrups, a cough that has been going on for more than eight weeks should be taken seriously.

Nearly one out of every ten Americans sees a doctor every year because of cough. This means plenty of people do make their way to the doctor seeking treatment for disruptive hacking. What statistics don't show is how many people emerge after their doctor's visit (or several doctors' visits) symptom free. I've had numerous patients whose cough has led them on a wild-goose chase for relief. They've seen multiple medical specialists, undergone numerous tests for conditions such as allergies and asthma, and even received chest X-rays. Yet they're still dealing with a chronic cough.

Usually, when they land in my office and I ask if they've been checked for acid reflux, they're incredulous: "Why would I be? I don't have heartburn." (Unlike you, they haven't read this book and discovered that the absence of heartburn doesn't mean absence of acid damage.) When chronic cough is present, an exam often reveals swelling of the vocal cords and/or larynx and a general sort of thickening of the tissues of the throat. These are the telltale signs that "acid was here."

After I realized the frustration chronic cough had caused for so many of my patients, I designed Dr. Aviv's Chronic Cough Algorithm. This diagnostic flow chart is designed to help get you relief faster. You will find the complete cough algorithm in the accompanying figure, but I'll share the critical first step with you here: if you smoke, stop. It doesn't matter what you smoke or how you smoke it—cigarettes, cigars, marijuana—whatever it is, you must stop completely. That goes for vaping, too. There's no healthy way to inhale tobacco carcinogens, even if it's just a "social" habit. Smoking marijuana isn't any better, which I'll explain in greater depth in chapter 6.

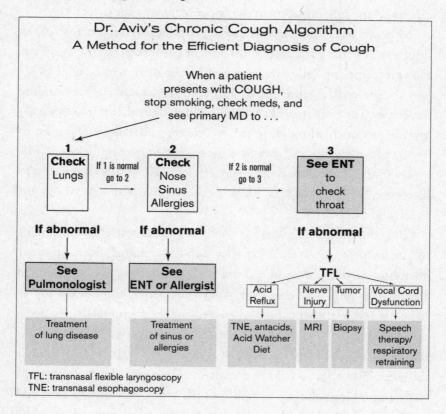

Dr. Aviv's Chronic Cough Algorithm
A Method for the Efficient Diagnosis of Cough

When a patient presents with COUGH, stop smoking, check meds, and see primary MD to . . .

1
Check Lungs

If 1 is normal go to 2

2
Check Nose Sinus Allergies

If 2 is normal go to 3

3
See ENT to check throat

If abnormal

See Pulmonologist

Treatment of lung disease

If abnormal

See ENT or Allergist

Treatment of sinus or allergies

If abnormal

TFL

Acid Reflux

Nerve Injury

Tumor

Vocal Cord Dysfunction

TNE, antacids, Acid Watcher Diet

MRI

Biopsy

Speech therapy/ respiratory retraining

TFL: transnasal flexible laryngoscopy
TNE: transnasal esophagoscopy

From Symptoms to Diagnosis: Getting Checked for Throatburn Reflux

When you present persistent throat-related symptoms to an otolaryngologist (an ENT doctor), they are going to want to take a look at your throat. I'm not just talking about the "stick out your tongue" test, although this can reveal any inflammation in the upper regions of the throat.

More detailed throat exams used to require sedation because of the difficulty in getting any sort of instrument past the powerful gag reflex. However, an exam called the transnasal flexible laryngoscopy (TFL) is now the preferred method for viewing your larynx and the surrounding structures. The brilliance of any transnasal exam is that it involves passing an instrument through your nose, thereby allowing a physician to bypass the gag reflex and view the tissues and structures below. While it may sound unpleasant to have any sort of "instrument" inserted into your nose, the tool used is as thin as a cooked piece of spaghetti, and just as soft and flexible, too.

The miniature TFL camera at the tip of this maneuverable spaghetti-like instrument is connected to a television-like monitor that allows your doctor to see your throat in real time. What will typically be examined are the vocal folds—do they look swollen and red, likely to be the source of hoarseness or throat pain? Is there evidence of postnasal drip or accumulated mucus, the possible cause of chronic cough or a lumplike sensation in the throat? I find the most powerful aspect of this type of exam is the patient's connection to the experience. Since no sedation is required (only a numbing solution sprayed into the nose), patients are alert and awake during the procedure and can directly see the effects of acidic foods and beverages.

I've performed TFL on thousands of people, and the procedure has allowed me to reveal to frustrated patients the sources of their nagging and uncomfortable symptoms: not only what comes up, but what comes down, meaning *both* refluxed gastric acid and frankly acidic material coming down from the mouth. Most who hear this are perplexed by the revelation. You know by now that symptoms of throatburn reflux without the presence of heartburn can indicate a more severe level of acid damage, often due to everyday habits that include consumption of substances that both loosen the LES and increase stomach acid production (coffee, chocolate), and substances that are directly acidic like soda and certain types of alcohol. Fun fact: Coffee and chocolate are actually not very acidic, but their physiological properties make them harmful for people with acid reflux. The methylxanthine in coffee and chocolate loosens the LES and increases hydrochloric acid production by the stomach.

What happens after a diagnosis of throatburn reflux depends on how severe the visible acid damage is and how long the symptoms have been occurring. There are other considerations, as the next steps are based on each patient's dietary habits, lifestyle, and overall health, but these are the two main factors at play. In all cases, nothing is more critical to tissue healing than the elimination of the acidic substances that are responsible for the damage. Some patients will also be given specific lifestyle adjustments, such as increasing the time between meals and sleep (at least three hours) or establishing dedicated periods of vocal rest, vital for recovering singers, radio DJs, and other vocal performers. Others will be given a dose of an acid-reducing or acid-weakening medication to accelerate healing.

The care and concern for a person who has throatburn reflux does not end here, as there is still the critical matter of esophageal health and the potential for a precancerous or cancerous condition to exist. Comprehensive treatment must include a follow-up exam of the esophagus, which can be done in a matter of minutes in your ENT's or even gastroenterologist's office with a transnasal esophagoscopy (TNE). Unfortunately, not every patient will be given the option of this test and may have to ask about it themselves—but if progress finally has its way, that's about to change.

The Evolution of the Esophageal Exam

In the early 1900s, a renowned American otolaryngologist, Dr. Chevalier Jackson, pioneered a method for examining the esophagus with a rigid, two-foot-long, hollow, stainless steel rod about the width of your thumb. This test, referred to as the rigid endoscopy, was performed on conscious patients who were lying flat on their back. You can imagine how unpleasant this experience was for patients *and* doctors, the latter of which no doubt had to struggle with a squirming, writhing individual while trying to assess the state of their esophagus.

Fast-forward more than a hundred years and you'll discover that this type of test is still being performed, although now it will only be done in an operating room with the patient under general anesthesia. In current practice, *rigid esophagoscopy* is rarely used to diagnose reflux disease; its primary use is to rule out cancer of the esophagus and to remove ingested foreign bodies. The procedure requires general anesthesia, which has a series of known risks, including stroke, heart attack, heart rhythm problems, and drops in blood pressure.

As a result of the risks of rigid esophagoscopy under general anesthesia, flexible cameras have been developed that allow examination of the esophagus using either light sedation or no sedation at all. These flexible cameras are employed in two different types of esophageal exams, upper endoscopy or esophagogastroduodenoscopy (EGD) and transnasal esophagoscopy (TNE). When someone is suspected of having acid reflux disease and related precancerous or cancerous conditions, more often than not they will be instructed to get an EGD, despite the viable and usually safer alternative of the TNE. Let's look at these two types of tests further and explore especially the marked differences between them.

In **upper endoscopy,** which is performed trans-orally, a small camera is used to examine the esophagus, stomach, and duodenum (the upper portion of the small intestine right below the stomach). Lower endoscopy is otherwise known as colonoscopy. Upper endoscopy is almost always performed with the patient under a type of sedation known as "twilight" anesthesia or intravenous conscious sedation. This is when the medication administered through the veins allows the patient to sleep through the procedure. The procedure can be worrisome for some patients because the medication that is used for this kind of sedation is known to have side effects that include a risk of "cardiopulmonary unplanned events"—medical-speak for respiratory arrest, stroke, and heart attack. The risk is small but finite, occurring in roughly 0.5 percent of patients undergoing the procedure. Although some experience complications, few die as a result, but the numbers are large enough to scare patients away from an examination they may desperately need.

In August 2014, upper endoscopy received some unwanted publicity with the death of comedian Joan Rivers, who experienced an untoward medical event when she underwent a sedated upper endoscopy and succumbed to it several days later. While we don't know what exactly transpired during Ms. Rivers's procedure, this preventable tragic event raised awareness that there are alternatives to sedation when a patient requires an upper endoscopy. In some cases, sedation is an unavoidable path to diagnosing and therefore devising treatment for a medical problem. But when it comes to the esophagus, this isn't the case.

A less costly and less risky option that has been around since the 1990s is the **transnasal esophagoscopy,** which I helped pioneer. This procedure allows for the esophagus to be examined without sedation other than some numbing medication misted into the nose. Because this test is performed through the nose—just like the transnasal laryngoscopy (TFL), which you read about earlier—there is zero need for sedation. It can be performed with the patient wide awake, sitting upright in a chair in a doctor's office, and it takes only minutes to perform. When the exam is over, the patient can get up and walk right out of the office and resume their day. Other than a nosebleed, there are no known risks. It is much safer for the patient and costs much less.

Use of TNE is standard in my practice, and it's the technique that I've been using for years. Not only does it eliminate the risks involved with anesthesia, it is as effective as the so-called conventional tests in identifying evidence of tissue damage in the esophagus, whether it's inflammation, Barrett's esophagus, or esophageal cancer (although the latter two require biopsies for diagnosis).

Another Reason That TNE Is Safer Than Traditional Upper Endoscopy

Cross-contamination is a known risk in medical procedures, and in 2013, Senator Patty Murray of Washington released a scathing report on patient safety during endoscopy due to cross-contamination that occurs when potentially infectious material, bacteria, fungus, and viruses are inadvertently transmitted from one patient to another through the instrument used to examine the patient. This problem is particular to the camera attached to the endoscopy instrument that carries scopes with special channels. These are tunnel-like pathways within the scope that allow for passage of instruments for performing biopsy. This channel-carrying scope has a complex series of nooks and crannies where bacteria can hide. The good news with TNE is that the scope used doesn't carry the biopsy channel, so there is no place for the potentially infectious material to hide.

As I mentioned, if you're a current candidate for esophageal exam, you are more likely to have a physician suggest you get an upper endoscopy. However, thanks to the most recent American College of Gastroenterology's *Clinical Guideline: Diagnosis and Management of Barrett's Esophagus*, the tide seems to be turning in favor of TNE—a shift that will greatly benefit patients and practitioners interested in safer, less costly procedures. In the report, published in November 2015, the TNE was listed as "an alternative to conventional upper endoscopy for Barrett's esophagus screening." This official level of endorsement to gastroenterologists across the United States will help make TNE a more widely used and accepted method for examining the esophagus. If it is not offered to you, you can ask your physician about it. Patients deserve to be aware of all the options and should work with their physicians to reach a conclusion on what method would serve them best.

Dollars and Cents in the Medical Procedure Equation

With revenue of about $30 billion per year, upper endoscopy is a big business. With ten million procedures performed each year in the United States and growing at a rate of about 6 percent per year, the question of associated cost to the healthcare industry has been and will continue to be a factor in discussion about how to diagnose, prevent, and treat precancerous and cancerous conditions of the esophagus. As of this writing, the traditional, sedated endoscopy costs about $3,000. The physician's fee is about $200 per procedure, with the remaining costs going toward the facility where the procedure is performed. Naturally, facility owners and managers and medical device equipment companies have a strong disincentive to see a safer, less expensive option such as TNE promoted. Over the last twenty years, numerous studies and textbooks on TNE have been published, yet not only the public but some physicians are unaware of this alternative to traditional upper endoscopy that will accomplish as truthful an analysis of what is going on in the esophagus, stomach, and duodenum as the traditional upper endoscopy.

An unsedated exam such as TNE doesn't require the more expensive facilities, devices, and techniques that sedated exams do, and it provides the same information at a substantially lower cost to the economy, the healthcare industry, and individuals. For patients, there are nonmedical, financial benefits to considering TNE as an alternative to the traditional endoscopy. Because there is no sedation and the procedure takes twenty minutes to perform, they don't have to lose a day's work, which will cut down the ten million workdays lost to five million. So another way of looking at TNE is that it saves the economy the productivity of five million workdays.

I estimate, conservatively, that over half of the sedated endoscopies performed annually can be performed in a physician's office without sedation, eliminating risk to the patient and saving the health industry over $15 billion per year. Some patients have reservations about having a tiny camera in their nose (which is exceedingly safe); others fear sedation under any circumstances, thus disqualifying themselves from the traditional endoscopy. Still, patients deserve to be aware of all the options available to them.

The Role of Prescription and Over-the-Counter Medications in Treating Reflux Symptoms

An exam at your doctor's office could result in a variety of treatment plans, which will depend on the severity and duration of your symptoms. Treatment should undoubtedly include awareness and elimination (even just temporarily) of sources of dietary acid. Following a high-fiber, low-acid diet is not only the most powerful prescription for curbing acid damage, it is also essential for true healing and prevention. However, because symptoms often stem from decades of exposure to inflammatory foods, the damage cannot be reversed after just a few days of strategic, low-acid modifications to your diet; in other words, the recovery process can take time: 28 days is the minimal time needed to heal acid-damaged tissue. In many cases, the discomfort and pain of acid injury can be strong and persistent enough for you to seek more immediate relief than a diet can realistically offer, and this is where medication can play a role.

As a doctor, I am not against medicine—either over-the-counter or prescription—but when it comes to acid injury treatment, I urge my patients to be careful. With a precancerous condition such as Barrett's esophagus, a prescription medication is often a must to help accelerate healing and reduce risk for further damage.

Like aluminum-containing antacids, most medications have some type of side effect, even if it's one that won't be immediately revealed.

With prescription acid-reducing medication, the expectation is that your doctor has judged that the benefit to you is greater than the risk of side effects. I hope that you are receiving such informed and attentive care, but I also continue to encourage you to be an empowered patient—ask about alternatives with fewer side effects and inquire how long you'll need to be on the medication, since you know it's not a permanent solution. If dietary modifications aren't recommended, ask for nutritional guidance, or rely on the comprehensive low-acid plan you'll find in part III of this book. Not only using food as medicine, but thinking that *food is medicine,* is paramount to treating and preventing disease, and the singular benefit of a culinary cure is the absence of side effects.

In my own practice, patients with moderate to severe throatburn and/or heartburn symptoms are offered, in addition to dietary and lifestyle management, a prescription for a proton pump inhibitor (PPI), the most powerful class of antacid medications; a single dose can suppress stomach acid production for up to sixteen hours. When stomach acid is reduced, inflammation in the esophagus, throat, and surrounding areas can begin to heal. The problem with PPIs is that they require specific administration to be effective, and studies have revealed that 80 percent of Americans may be taking these powerful meds incorrectly. There are two steps to taking a PPI the correct way:

1. Take a PPI dose thirty to sixty minutes before you eat either breakfast or dinner, or both (allowing it to enter your bloodstream).

2. Eat something to "activate" the PPI within thirty to sixty minutes after taking the medication.

Even with the proper use of PPIs and/or other acid-reducing medications, recovery from acid damage can take time. In my practice, only 25 percent of patients with throatburn reflux symptoms improve after six weeks of treatment with PPIs, with a larger percentage experiencing relief after twelve weeks of use. Others will require medication for six months or longer before they begin to feel better. This is not to discourage you but rather to help you understand that there is no "magic pill" that will alleviate the symptoms caused by refluxed acid *and* promote rapid healing of tissues within the esophagus and throat that have been damaged, often by years of acid exposure.

The Danish Controversy: Are PPIs Safe?

When a Danish study came out in May 2014 concluding that regular, long-term use of certain PPIs was linked to greater risk of developing esophageal cancer, the use of this popular acid-blocking medication was put into question. It was an alarming argument, but it's not one you should give too much credence. The authors of the study were unable to control for significant risk factors for the development of esophageal cancer such as alcohol consumption. Nor were other lifestyle considerations, such as smoking or dietary habits, taken into consideration. Furthermore, numerous studies have suggested that PPIs may give a protective effect against both the precursor to esophageal cancer and esophageal cancer itself.

Now, if long-term PPI use has overlapped with persistent symptoms of throatburn and *waning* GERD symptoms that have been present for ten or more years, the risk for severe damage to esophageal tissue increases. If you or someone you know fits this patient profile, it's critical that an ENT or GI specialist see you as soon as possible.

Recovery from acid damage can take patience and consistency, but careful attention to medication use (if necessary) and a commitment to low-acid eating are guaranteed to reward you with good health. Not only will you finally be free of the nagging, disruptive, and painful symptoms caused by refluxed acid, you will also have significantly reduced your risk for developing the nation's fastest-growing form of cancer.

Now, without further delay, let's get to the part you've been waiting for: the dietary blueprint essential to healing and eliminating your acid-related symptoms.

PART II

Food and Lifestyle Prescriptions

CHAPTER 5

Understanding the Role of Proteins, Carbohydrates, and Fats in Healing Dietary Acid Damage

created the Acid Watcher Diet in response to the alarming trends tracking from the standard American diet, which is high in processed food, additives, acid, fats, sugar, and salt. The primary goal of the program is to use food to heal acid damage in the gastrointestinal region, reduce systemic and pepsin-driven inflammation, and help prevent an array of chronic diseases without vitamin deficiency, loss of energy, or waist-busting sugar or salt cravings. While highly acidic foods—processed and natural—had to be ditched in order to attain this goal, I didn't want the Acid Watcher Diet to be just a diet of ruthless elimination; on the contrary, I wanted to see my patients expand their palates and options for satisfying and varied meals. That is the reason I designed the plan around three dietary pillars: consumption of high-quality macronutrients, high concentration of fiber, and replacing high-acid foods with low-acid foods. Before we delve into the day-by-day planning, it will be helpful to review a few basics about nutrition.

The Acid Watcher's Guide to Macronutrients

The food we consume is a source of the many *macronutrients* and *micronutrients* our body needs to remain alive. Macronutrients are *proteins, carbohydrates,* and *fats*—the structural, caloric components that create energy. Micronutrients are *minerals, vitamins,* and *phytochemicals,* compounds that regulate the body's functions, fight free radicals that create oxidative stress, and repair cellular damage. *Minerals,* which are derived from plant-based foods, build up our tissue and maintain organ health and pH balance throughout the body. *Vitamins* provide additional antioxidants to help enzymes already present in your body to fight inflammation. *Phytochemicals,* which give plants their distinct color, taste, smell, and texture, fight inflammation and are crucial to the prevention of certain diseases, including cancer.

Macronutrients are a rich source for micronutrients, and under ideal conditions, a macronutrient-balanced diet gives your body all the nutrients it needs to function optimally.

Despite their crucial role in supplying nutrients essential to maintaining our general health, the three macronutrients—proteins, carbohydrates, and fats—have taken their turns as punching bags in a zealous battle against the bulge. Unfortunately, this well-intentioned quest has given rise to medically questionable diet fads. We've had the trend of a low-fat diet replaced by a low-carb diet, then taken over by a high-protein diet before the cycle started all over again.

I believe that diets that deprive your body of any of the three macronutrients are never optimal for your health in the long run. If you are omitting an entire macronutrient—whether protein, fat, or carbohydrate—you are eliminating the vitamins, minerals, phytochemicals, and other compounds that reduce oxidative stress and inflammation and keep your hormones in balance. For an Acid Watcher, it is also important to remember that each macronutrient helps, in its own way, to maintain and repair cellular functions, especially in the delicate tissue of your esophagus. So a balanced diet is essential to your health.

Macronutrient-depletion diets are also unsustainable in the long run, as they either leave you famished (especially if you give up fiber), energy deficient (low-carb, low-protein), and/or with unregulated moods (low-fat). Scientific evidence suggests that when a macronutrient is removed from the diet to attain weight loss—as in removing carbohydrates from a high-protein diet—the effect is only short term and in the long term, it may ultimately lead to weight gain.

There is no evidence to suggest that macronutrient depletion can help reduce acid damage to the esophagus or other organs in the aerodigestive tract. Only an increase in dietary fiber intake will help extinguish the internal fires lit by acid damage by lessening inflammatory pepsin triggers, improving digestion, and reducing cravings for salty, sugary, and acidic foods. I will discuss, in more detail, the crucial role of dietary fiber in the next chapter.

AN ACID WATCHER'S GUIDE TO PROTEINS

Protein is a crucial macronutrient that helps your body grow and repair itself. This is particularly important for most acid reflux patients who have inflamed or damaged tissue in the esophagus or throat. Amino acids found in proteins will aid in the reconstruction of these cells and tissues. Other important chemicals in our body, such as hormones and enzymes that help regulate digestion, are also made up of protein, and anything that can help with digestion should be a crucial component in a diet that combats inflammation and acid damage.

As you may have surmised by now, anything that can help with digestion is a crucial benefit to people with acid reflux disease. In the case of protein, it's not just a question of having enough protein but the *type* of protein as well.

When you choose your protein source, consider the overall nutritional value. Some sources of protein, such as red meat, are high in saturated fat. Excessive amounts of fat can exacerbate acid reflux by impairing the ability of the lower esophageal sphincter (LES) to function optimally. This can lead to stomach acid flowing unimpeded up and out of the stomach, where it can injure the esophagus. So if you are an Acid Watcher, I recommend staying away from red meat—but not from all animal-derived proteins.

There are two sources of healthy protein—*animal* and *vegetable*. Animal-derived proteins that are good for Acid Watchers include sardines, salmon, tuna, halibut, turkey (light meat, no skin), chicken (light meat, no skin), yogurt, kefir, and eggs. Examples of vegetable-derived proteins include peanuts, oatmeal, cashews, beans (all types), tofu, edamame, walnuts, soy milk (non–genetically modified), hazelnuts, whole grains, quinoa, broccoli, spinach, kale, and spirulina.

What Is a Genetically Modified Organism?

You may know a few basics about genetic engineering, a relatively new branch of science conceived and developed with the noble intention of preventing and eliminating disease, hunger, and other persistent challenges facing humanity. The idea is that by manipulating certain parts of the genome in any living thing—as in our flora and fauna—we may be able to reduce the genetic risk for life-threatening disease like cancer in humans, or improve the quantity of plant-based foods by increasing crop resistance to harmful agents like pests. In short, we can live longer, healthier lives and grow food that is plentiful and sturdy enough to feed the ever-expanding population. At least that's the theory. In practice we really don't know the long-term impact of modifying the genome in plants or animals. Our food products are especially vulnerable to unforeseen effects of biochemical changes that genome alteration requires. For example, whatever extends the shelf life of a fruit or vegetable may be harmful to our bodies if we consume it. I believe that until we have more information on the effects of genetic modification, it is safer to stay away from all genetically modified food products.

Beans and eggs, especially egg yolks, can be hard for some people to digest. I recommend that they be consumed in moderation. For best results, animal sources of protein should primarily be eaten in combination with vegetables, ideally prepared raw or steamed, for easier digestion.

Why You Should Choose Organic Meat and Poultry

Processed foods are not limited to products that are acidified, bottled, or jarred. Animals raised on most feedlots in the United States typically spend their lives sun-deprived and are fed excessive amounts of grains riddled with pesticide residue, antibiotics, and growth hormones—all artificial additives. These practices diminish the potential for animal-based products to have beneficial properties, such as providing vitamins E and B and beta-carotene, and instead introduce higher levels of omega-6 fatty acids and caustic chemical debris, both of which can contribute to inflammation. This is why I recommend that whenever you eat eggs, dairy, or meat, it should ideally be organic and come from a grass-fed animal.

CARBOHYDRATES—WHY WE NEED THEM

Diets that have tried to regulate the intake of carbohydrates have come and gone. But one thing we know for sure—carbs remain an essential source of energy for your brain, muscles, and heart. Based on their molecular structure, carbohydrates are divided into two groups: complex carbs and simple carbs.

Complex (Good) Carbs

Complex carbohydrates are broken down into sugar gradually over a longer period of time because of their more complex molecular structure, which is different from that of simple carbohydrates. This allows for a slow, gradual release of sugar into the bloodstream, providing the body with a steady, more balanced source of energy. After a person consumes complex carbs, blood sugar levels should remain relatively stable.

Here are natural sources of common complex (good) carbohydrates:

Vegetables: Broccoli, cucumber, cauliflower, spinach, potatoes, corn, carrots, lettuce

Whole grains: Brown rice, oats, whole-grain cereal, whole-wheat pasta, whole-wheat bread, whole-grain bread

Legumes: Beans (all kinds)

Fruit: Apricots, apples, pears, prunes, oranges, grapefruit, plums

Dairy: Milk, cheese, yogurt (in limited amounts)

What is crucial for an Acid Watcher to remember, however, is that while most of these foods have a high pH value, some of them—like oranges, grapefruit, and prunes—are extremely acidic and should be avoided by people with acid reflux. In chapter 9, we will focus more on the pH-friendly but acid-reflux-deadly foods.

Simple (Bad) Carbs

As their name suggests, simple carbs have a much simpler molecular structure than complex carbs. For that reason, they get broken down into sugar very rapidly, often causing drastic sugar spikes in the blood.

Simple carbs form the foundation of most processed or commercially baked goods, such as cookies, doughnuts, chocolate, potato chips, and sugary soda, as well as thousands of other packaged foods we eat daily. In fact, almost all prepackaged foods, juices, sweeteners, "low-fat" foods, "low-calorie" foods, and most foods made with white flour, such as white pasta and white bread, contain simple carbs.

Consuming an excessive amount of simple carbs, especially from processed and refined foods devoid of fiber, instead of fueling the body with energy, will actually leave you feeling deprived. For example, eating a large piece of chocolate cake on an empty stomach will result in an immediate burst of energy, but just fifteen minutes to couple of hours later (depending on your metabolism), a wave of fatigue will settle in. What actually happens when an excessive amount of sugar rapidly reaches the blood? The pancreas starts producing large amounts of insulin until the blood sugar level drops. Once the blood sugar level drops, you often start feeling tired, which can lead to a craving of even more sugar. Then you reach for the ice cream sitting in the freezer, and the process starts all over again.

This is dangerous because unchecked sugar cravings over time can predispose you not only to acid reflux disease, but to obesity, type 2 diabetes, heart disease, and other physical maladies that plague so many of us living on a Western diet.

Here are some common simple carbs that should be avoided:

Fruit juices

Soft drinks

Table sugar

Cakes

Cookies (packaged or otherwise)

Candy

White bread

White pasta

Ice cream

Anything that contains high-fructose corn syrup

Many fruits such as bananas, mangoes, pomegranates, and raisins contain naturally occurring simple carbs, but that doesn't mean they should be avoided. They contain fiber and a wide variety of vitamins and minerals that your body needs. However, proceed with caution when it comes to fruit juices, even naturally squeezed, as they contain little or no fiber. The sugar reaches your bloodstream a lot faster, causing an unhealthy sugar spike.

Eating the right kind of carbs can ensure steady blood sugar levels. Balanced blood sugar correlates to steady energy and stifled cravings and quells overeating. Complex carbohydrates—vegetables, whole grains, dairy, legumes, and fruits—can keep blood sugar stable and prevent cravings, thereby optimizing weight-loss potential. Fruits and vegetables contain fiber and a wide variety of vitamins and minerals that your body needs to stay stable, energized, and acid free. So *increase* their

Do You Experience Bloating and Indigestion? These Carbs Could Be to Blame

Not all foods that are more alkaline are necessarily acid neutral. Onions and garlic, for example are not acidic, but they do play a role in bloating, indigestion, and heartburn. These foods are known as *fructans*, and they are part of the FODMAP group of carbohydrates. FODMAP stands for *fermentable, oligo-, di-, and monosaccharides, and polyols,* and was coined to describe a previously unrelated group of short-chain carbohydrates and sugar alcohols (polyols) that have three common functional properties. These substances can:

- *be poorly absorbed in the small intestine* and cause gas and bloating.

- *have a laxative effect,* thanks to their ability to essentially suck water into the intestines. This is especially true for fructans such as onion and garlic.

- *get rapidly fermented by bacteria:* Most FODMAPs, such as oligosaccharides and sugars, are short-chain carbs, which are rapidly fermented, leading to increased gas production.

intake. Berries and citrus—while micronutrient rich—are too acidic for people with acid damage. Their intake should be *reduced* in the Healing Phase of the diet and *managed* carefully in the Maintenance Phase. Simple carbohydrates—white bread and pastas and sugary drinks that contain high-fructose corn syrup—stimulate insulin production, causing sugar and acid spikes. *Eliminate* these carbohydrates from your diet for better overall health.

AN ACID WATCHER'S GUIDE TO FATS

Fat is one of the most crucial components of the human body. A healthy body is made up of 20 percent fat, with our brain being made up of

60 percent fat. Fat helps regulate our body temperature and protects internal organs from impact injury. It is also important for maintaining healthy levels of hormone production and joint lubrication. In addition, fat helps keep our nerve structure in place, which is crucial for neural transmission. Many essential vitamins and minerals are absorbed by our bodies only if they are attached to fat.

As an Acid Watcher, you will learn to replace *bad* fats with *good* fats. Bad fats are trans fats and (in excessive amounts) saturated fats. Good fats are unsaturated fats, which include monounsaturated fats and polyunsaturated fats. Let's get the bad out of the way first.

Trans Fats (Bad Fats)

Trans fat should absolutely be avoided by anyone with acid reflux disease. In fact, trans fat should be avoided by everyone. Most trans fats that make it onto our plates are formed during the processing of food in order to turn fat into a solid, as well as to make our processed food last longer. Ever wonder why that box of crackers you bought during the Bush administration is still so crispy and fresh? Thank you, trans fat.

Trans fat is formed when hydrogen ions are blasted into vegetable oil under pressure to make the fat stiffer. As a result, trans fat also goes under the catch-all name "hydrogenated oil." Cookies, potato chips, microwave popcorn, and most "healthy" butterlike substances like margarine that were wrongly embraced in the 1970s as a "healthy" alternative for butter are examples of trans fat in a pretty package.

Trans fat is bad for several reasons. It increases LDL levels (remember: that's the "bad" cholesterol), while at the same time decreasing HDL, high-density lipoprotein, known as the "good cholesterol" levels. This significantly increases our risk for heart disease. In addition, for people with acid reflux, trans fat loosens the lower esophageal sphincter (LES) so stomach acid can freely splash back up into the esophagus.

Saturated Fats

Saturated fat can be found in both animals and vegetables. The fatty layer under your skin that regulates your body temperature consists of saturated fat. The plaque in your arteries is also made up of saturated fat.

What usually makes saturated fat harmful to our health is not just the processing it often undergoes before reaching our dinner table, but the sheer amount of it that we eat. If you eat steak, you know that even a small portion takes a disproportionately large space on our plate. And, if like most Americans you follow a typical Western diet, you are probably having an animal protein for lunch, dinner, and in some cases, even breakfast. It shouldn't surprise you, therefore, that a diet high in saturated fat is often a major contributor to acid reflux disease.

If you don't have access to organic animal products, try to replace them with fats found in plants (avocado, coconut, olives, nuts, seeds), or the healthy fats found in fish, discussed in the following sections. Although saturated fat is needed in our bodies, excessive amounts are harmful. One of the most important points to remember regarding our food intake is that moderation does not mean "midway," as in 50/50. In the case of saturated fat, if you really want a percentage-type guide to follow, do not allow more than 10 percent of your daily fat intake to come from saturated fat. This is one of the reasons that the Acid Watcher Diet calls for you to eat either a vegetarian lunch or dinner every day. You will automatically reduce the amount of saturated fats consumed daily while increasing your fiber intake.

Unsaturated Fats (Good Fats)

MONOUNSATURATED FATS: Monounsaturated fats are considered a good type of fat when consumed in moderation. They help increase our body's HDL levels while lowering LDL levels. These fats are liquid at room temperature but solidify when refrigerated. They're found in a wide variety of foods, such as meat, whole milk, olives and olive oil, avocados, almonds, cashews, and peanuts. With the exception of red meat, mono-unsaturated fats are typically good choices for people with acid reflux disease.

However, a subset of monounsaturated fat is not good for those with acid reflux—vegetable oils made from seeds. Examples include soybean oil, corn oil, canola oil, safflower oil, cottonseed oil, grapeseed oil, and sunflower oil. These seed oils usually require high-tech processing using extreme heat, pressure, and/or chemical solvents in order for the oil to be extracted. High heat destabilizes the molecular structure of these oils, resulting in free radical formation, which is highly inflammatory and caustic to the body.

Cold-pressed vegetable oils are always the best option for people with acid reflux. If possible, choose extra virgin olive oil, which is oil that was extracted from the first pressing of the olive fruit. Additional pressings produce oil of a lesser quality. If you've ever had a chance to smell and taste homemade olive oil, you know that it has a distinct and strong scent. Olive oil without a scent has probably been heavily processed or deodorized and should be avoided.

The best sources of monounsaturated fat for people with acid reflux are the following:

Cold-pressed extra virgin olive oil

Avocado and avocado oil

Coconut oil

Cashews

Almonds

Peanuts

POLYUNSATURATED FATS (OMEGA-3 AND OMEGA-6): Polyunsaturated fat is one of the healthiest forms of fat. Two of the more important subcategories of polyunsaturated fat are omega-3 and omega-6 fats. They are considered essential fats because they cannot be produced by our bodies and must be obtained through the consumption of food.

Omega-3 is produced in the leafy parts of the plant during photosynthesis. Omega-6 is produced predominantly in the seeds of plants. Animals acquire the largest amount of omega-3 fats by directly consuming leafy plants or grass. That is why meat or eggs from grass-fed animals will have more omega-3 than from grain-fed animals.

Fish is a potent source of omega-3 fat. Fish acquire their omega-3 from eating algae or plankton naturally found in the ocean. However, not all fish are created equal. Just as with land animals allowed to run free and eat grass for their sustenance, wild fish are richer in omega-3 than farmed fish. In addition, cold-water fish have the highest amount of omega-3 because their natural habitat promotes the best conditions for the accumulation of this type of fat in their bodies.

Omega-3 is considered one of the most beneficial types of fat as it helps maintain the integrity and permeability of our cell walls. It also helps metabolize glucose, lowers cholesterol, and supports brain function.

Omega-6 fatty acids are more complicated. They are naturally found in seeds, grains and nuts, and vegetable oils such as canola and sunflower oil. Certain types of omega-6 fats have undeniable health benefits, but the Western diet, which is characterized by a high intake of processed food rich in seed oils, has compromised their benefits.

Much research has been done trying to find the ideal ratio between omega-6 and omega-3 consumption, but I think it is difficult for anyone who is not a scientist to fully understand what these numbers mean in a practical sense. Therefore, I would like to simplify this with a take-home message—remove processed and deep-fried foods from your diet. Both are acid forming; the latter are certainly fattening. At the same time, increase your fish intake to at least twice a week and eat plenty of vegetables so your body will find a natural balance between omega-6 and omega-3 fat.

Here are some healthy polyunsaturated fats:

Omega-3-Rich Foods

Salmon	Halibut	Kale
Anchovies	Tuna	Seaweed
Herring	Eggs (from grass-fed chickens)	Flaxseed
Mackerel		Walnuts
Trout	Spinach	Marine algae
Sardine		

Omega-6-Rich Foods

Sunflower seeds	Eggs	Pecans
Pumpkin seeds	Avocados	Cashews
Poultry	Walnuts	

HOW "LOW FAT" CAN BE BAD FOR YOU

It seems that the ongoing crusade to promote and consume low-fat items has failed to make us a healthy and slim nation. Perhaps with our best intentions, we continue to mistake fat-free or low-fat items for healthy. It is obvious by now that this simply is not the case.

I was recently shopping for some plain yogurt and got distracted by the colorful labels on the fruit yogurts. All the available types, and there were plenty of them, were either fat-free or low-fat. I couldn't find a regular fruit yogurt anywhere. Now, you might be thinking, "What's wrong with that?" Well, it's flawed logic to think that by simply removing or decreasing one macronutrient from our diets, we can ultimately improve our overall health. Nature is a lot more complex than that. As I scanned the label of one of the fruit yogurts that is both highly praised and popular for its numerous health claims, I realized that its sugar content was 23 grams per 113 grams of yogurt. That's the equivalent of eating almost five teaspoons of pure sugar in one sitting, just as a snack! It's even more preposterous when you consider that yogurt is supposed to be healthy food.

At first, one might think that the yogurt labeled fat-free couldn't be that bad. After all, the fat was presumably removed from the yogurt. But that's actually where the problem lies. Fat gives us a sense of satiation, or the sense of feeling full. With fat-free food, we tend to eat a lot more. In a sense, we chase that sense of fullness, while ingesting excessive (and even harmful) amounts of sugar along the way.

Another important property of fat we need to consider is that it creates flavor. Without fat, food manufacturers have to add a lot of sugar and/or artificial flavors to make the yogurt tasty. Our overall national health will not improve by demonizing and expelling macronutrients from our food. Our health will only improve when we stop adding unnecessary artificial components to it.

Final Thoughts on Macronutrients and Micronutrients

Unfortunately, the industrialization of our food supply since the 1970s has affected our ability to get the proper amount of micronutrients to the table. Pesticides, overly acidic or basic soil, and food processing and preserving can all drastically reduce the nutritional value of food—the minerals, vitamins, and phytochemicals. Take a look at the ingredients printed on the packaging of products currently on your refrigerator or pantry shelves. How many words do you recognize as food as opposed to chemicals? How many can you pronounce? Remember that the longer the list of additives and preservatives and the more unpronounceable the words, the worse it is for your health.

The industrialized, processed food that you find in your local grocery store has been acidified, its pH has been lowered, and its micronutrient viability has been significantly reduced. Even cooking some plant-based foods—such as broccoli and zucchini—can strip them of certain anti-oxidants, such as vitamin C. This is why it's important to avoid processed foods and replace them with plenty of organic, minimally cooked fruits and vegetables (steaming is my preferred option). I also recommend that whenever you eat eggs, dairy, or meat, it should ideally be organic and come from a grass-fed animal to ensure that your diet is balanced in macronutrients and that you are getting all the micronutrients your body needs.

CHAPTER 6

The Fiber Gap and How to Bridge It

Consuming a high concentration of fiber is one of the three crucial components of the Acid Watcher Diet. You may wonder how fiber makes the cut in a diet designed to help produce relief and healing from the effects of acid reflux. The reasons are many: not only does fiber improve digestion—probably its most widely known benefit—but it has proven over time to be a multifaceted instrument of optimum health. Let's talk about the evolving understanding of fiber and the vital role it will play in your recovery from acid damage, and in your overall health, too.

The Facts About Fiber

Fiber has been on the radar of those interested in health for over 1,800 years. In AD 130, the Greek physician Galen wrote about foods that "excite the bowels to evacuate and those that prevent them," and how white breads were "sticky and slow" and brown breads were "good for the bowels." Centuries later a man whose last name you'll recognize, Dr. J. H. Kellogg, would prescribe high-fiber wheat bran to those visiting his sanitarium, and in 1915, his brand would introduce the first high-fiber cereal, Bran Flakes. Later, in the 1940s, this good-for-digestion foodstuff was finally given the term of "dietary fiber."

Dietary fiber was first defined as the nondigestible part of plants, specifically the outer wall of plant cells that create a plant's "skeleton." These walls consist mostly of cellulose, a complex carbohydrate that plants build to help protect against pests and other environmental assaults. This protective nature also helps cellulose remain mostly intact as it passes through the human digestive system; not even gastric acid or our most degradative digestive enzymes can break it, or other equally fibrous components, down completely. A perfect example of a cellulose-rich dietary fiber is bran, the hard outer layer that surrounds cereal grains such as wheat, rice, and barley (bran is what makes bread "brown," to refer back to Galen's observation).

Later research helped expand the definition of dietary fiber to include other plant-based materials that were less resistant to digestion but still were never fully broken down after passing through the digestive tract. This included substances such as pectin, found in beets, apples, and fruit peels; lignins, found in radishes, spinach, and kale; and oligosaccharides, such as inulin, which occurs naturally in leeks, onion, and asparagus. These two different fiber types varying in digestibility are divided into two categories: soluble and insoluble fiber.

Soluble fiber attracts water and forms a gel-like consistency during digestion. This helps slow down the digestive process and increase feelings of fullness. Food sources include beans, lentils, nuts, seeds, oat bran, pears, Brussels sprouts, and sweet potatoes.

Insoluble fiber does not attract or absorb water and instead works like a stiff broom sweeping out the intestines as the insoluble fiber passes through your digestive tract. In this way, it can help cleanse the colon and combat constipation. Sources of insoluble fiber include wheat bran, whole grains, dark leafy vegetables, broccoli, cabbage, and zucchini.

While some foods have more of one type of fiber over the other, most whole fruits, vegetables, nuts, and seeds contain both insoluble and soluble fiber. For this reason, as an Acid Watcher, you'll simply want to increase your overall fiber intake rather than try to eat more of one specific type. According to the American Dietetic Association, you should be eating 25 to 35 grams a day, but if you're anything like the average American, you're eating closer to 15 grams of fiber a day. A 2014 review published in *Nutrition Journal* suggested that bridging this "fiber gap" is a critical component of improving overall health, not just in the United States but across the world.

The Top Ten Proven Benefits of Eating More Fiber

It's long been known that dietary fiber can improve digestion. Studies of early humans and contemporary African communities have connected diets high in fiber to larger bowel movements, which is typically a reflection of faster transit times (i.e., the movement of waste through the body) and optimized digestion. Conversely, low-weight bowel movements, the product of a fiber-poor diet, have been linked to increased risk of diverticular disease and bowel and colon cancers. Based on these observations, it may seem as though fiber is just a force that helps push things through our digestive tract. But it's proven to be and do much more than that.

A 2011 study conducted by researchers from the National Cancer Institute and published in the *Archives of Internal Medicine* found that dietary fiber intake was "significantly inversely associated with the risk of total death and death from CVD [cardiovascular disease], infectious diseases, and respiratory diseases in both men and women." In other words, eating more fiber could help you avoid disease and live longer, making it a critical factor in longevity.

While the study pointed out the importance of "cereal fiber," or grain-based fiber, a closer analysis provided by Lawrence de Koning and Frank Hu, both from the Harvard School of Public Health, suggested that it may not be cereal fiber that delivers, by itself, the health benefits for which it is credited. Instead, it could be the natural package of nutrients that comes with fiber—vitamins, minerals, and other phytonutrients ranging from antioxidants to zinc—that protects human tissues from damage.

Whether it's due to fiber's structural integrity, nutritional nature, or some other yet-to-be-discovered beneficial property, increasing your fiber intake during the Acid Watcher Diet and beyond will reward you in a number of ways. Some are specific to your recovery from the effects of refluxed acid, and others relate to improvements in your overall health. Here are the top ten proven benefits of eating more fiber:

10. **Lower cholesterol levels:** When soluble fiber turns into a gel-like substance during digestion, it becomes sticky and binds to bacteria and other free-floating substances. One of these substances is LDL cholesterol, which can be absorbed into the viscous vehicle as it makes its way through your digestive tract and excreted through waste. When you lower your LDL cholesterol and total cholesterol, you reduce your risk of developing heart disease, the number one killer in the United States.

9. **Lower heart disease risk:** Research has shown that heart disease risk is increasingly lowered for every additional 7 grams/day of fiber consumed. (To give you an idea of how much fiber this is, one cup of raspberries contains 8 grams of fiber; when added to almond milk in Dr. Aviv's Berry Smoothie Blast [page 158], you have a high-fiber smoothie that is very tasty as well.) The lowered disease risk could be due to the effects of fiber on cholesterol or other benefits, such as improved insulin sensitivity, and lowered blood pressure. No matter the mechanism, according to the 2004 study "Dietary Fiber and Risk of Coronary Heart Disease," eating a diet that's high in fiber-rich foods to prevent heart disease is "based on a wealth of consistent scientific evidence."

8. **Controlled blood sugar:** A diet that's high in refined carbohydrates—carbs that have been mostly stripped of their fiber—has been linked to hyperglycemia, the blood sugar disorder characterized by too much glucose in the bloodstream, and can be a precursor to type 2 diabetes. Conversely, fiber-rich complex carbohydrates have been shown to help control blood sugar by slowing the digestive process and balancing the blood sugar response. Because fiber doesn't trigger much of an insulin response, it can counter less-fibrous parts of a food that do trigger insulin (this is why you should always eat fruits and vegetables whole and with the peel,

when possible and especially when it's organic produce, which has peels that have not been compromised by pesticides). If you have type 2 diabetes, keeping your blood sugar balanced is an important part of staying healthy. In all people, balanced blood sugar is key to keeping cravings under control and preventing energy crashes.

7. **Relief for issues related to IBS, constipation, and other digestion woes:** Recall that dietary fiber has been shown to increase bowel movement size and accelerate transit time. These two benefits alone can be life changing for those who have IBS and/or chronic constipation. Larger, heavier stools cleanse the colon and produce relief within a backed-up digestive tract. A clean colon also lessens the chance of developing the painful condition of diverticulitis.

6. **Reduced pressure on the lower esophageal sphincter (LES):** When your digestive system isn't functioning properly, the pressure created by constipation, gas, or excess bloating can extend up to the LES and weaken the important closure that shuts gastric acid out from the tissues above. As fiber works to improve the efficiency and effectiveness of your digestive system, it will also help decrease the type of upward pressure that can open the door to acid damage.

5. **Improved gut health:** Oligosaccharides, found in many soluble fibers, resist digestion in the small intestine but go on to be fermented by gut bacteria in the colon. In this way, these fermentable fibers act as prebiotics that stimulate the production of beneficial bacteria, which are known to improve nutrient absorption, increase immunity, and lessen the presence of pathogenic bacteria. Artichokes, leeks, broccoli, wheat, oats, and soybeans are good sources of prebiotics.

4. **Assistance in weight loss and maintenance:** Increasing your fiber intake is one of the smartest, yet simplest ways to promote

weight loss. Foods with dietary fiber help you feel fuller faster and longer by slowing down digestion and, in the case of soluble fiber, expanding in volume, helping you feel satiated with smaller food volumes. Research shows that increasing your fiber intake can reduce the number of calories you consume. It may seem mathematically impossible to be able to increase what you eat and decrease your caloric intake, but that's the magic of fiber. Fiber itself contains no calories, which is why foods with a high proportion of fiber (broccoli, spinach, celery, and kale) are low in calories.

3. **Reduced inflammation:** Dietary fiber indirectly and directly helps diminish levels of inflammation. By mitigating inflammatory triggers, such as high blood sugar, bad intestinal bacteria, and high LDL cholesterol, it indirectly lowers inflammation throughout the body. The mechanisms behind fiber's more direct anti-inflammatory abilities aren't entirely clear yet, but there are a few plausible possibilities. For one, eating foods high in fiber has been associated with lower levels of inflammatory markers, such as C-reactive protein, which have known links to chronic inflammation. Dietary fiber also decreases lipid oxidation, which helps minimize the production of damage-instigating free radicals. Additionally, many fiber-rich foods are chock-full of antioxidants, nutrients, and minerals that counteract the effects of inflammation. Whole grains, for example, contain several minerals, including zinc and selenium, both of which have been proven to help lower levels of oxidative stress. The net result of this taming of inflammation through dietary fiber is a powerful protectant against infectious and respiratory diseases.

2. **Staving off the sparks of cancer:** We ingest carcinogens every day, whether we know it or not. Processed and charred meats, nonorganic produce (due to pesticide residue), and foods and drinks containing chemical additives are just a few of the ways carcinogens can be introduced to the body. The good news is that by increasing your fiber intake you can help rid your body of these

carcinogens before they cause any long-term damage. Fiber is believed to bind to carcinogens and other toxins and then promote the excretion of these materials as waste. Dietary fiber's sticky skill in this case helps reduce intestinal carcinogenesis, or the formation of cancer.

And the #1 benefit of increased fiber consumption for Acid Watchers . . .

1. **Reduced risk of Barrett's esophagus and esophageal cancer:** A meta-study published in the journal *Food Science and Nutrition* in October 2015 suggested that dietary fiber intake is "significantly associated with reduced risk of Barrett's esophagus and esophageal cancer." As an ENT who's seen too many lives disrupted by precancerous and frankly malignant tissue in the esophagus, I find this benefit of fiber exceptional and exciting; it's proof that how you eat each day can be health- and life-altering. The study went on to identify inositol hexaphosphate, a component found in high-fiber foods, as a factor in the cancer-fighting ring (at least within the esophagus). Inositol hexaphosphate has been shown to inhibit the growth rate of cancer cells in the esophagus by limiting their ability to multiply and stimulating cell death.

Bridging the Fiber Gap

As you can see, eating a diet rich in fiber is a good rule of thumb, whether you have acid reflux disease or not. As an Acid Watcher, increasing your fiber intake will be second only to eliminating acidic foods. If your diet currently only provides around 10 to 15 grams of fiber per day—the average intake for most Americans—you may be wondering how you'll go about essentially doubling this to reach the recommended amount of fiber of 25 to 35 grams. I've created two simple yet specific rules to help you achieve this increase:

Eat a daily minimum of 1 pound of vegetables above pH 5, half of which should be consumed raw

Vegetables are the triple threat of the food world: they're jam-packed with minerals and nutrients you won't find anywhere else, wildly low in calories (despite being deliciously filling), and full of fiber. While you'll find fiber in every single plant food, some contain more than others: artichokes, broccoli, carrots, and spinach are just a few of the veggies that are excellent sources of fiber.

To eat 1 pound of vegetables each day, 1/2 pound of which is cooked and 1/2 pound of which is eaten raw, you will need to consume about the equivalent of two cups of vegetables (measured when raw). Consuming both raw and cooked vegetables will help ensure that you get a greater variety of antioxidants. Some vegetables, such as carrots, asparagus, cabbage, mushrooms, and spinach, offer a greater concentration of antioxidants when cooked compared to when eaten raw (if they're prepared by steaming or boiling, that is). But you're likely to get more vitamin C from these foods if you eat them fresh out of the fridge. Broccoli is one nutritional powerhouse that you should try to eat raw, at least some of the time, as raw broccoli is higher in sulforaphane, a known anticarcinogen. The most important part of the vegetable rule is that you eat at least 1 pound of vegetables every day no matter how they're prepared, but do your best to eat 1/2 pound raw and 1/2 pound cooked.

In most cases, the easiest way to reach the daily intake goal of 1 pound of vegetables is to look beyond single sources. That is, you should enjoy a variety of vegetables with your meals. Take a look at the High-Fiber Salad (page 166) as an example. In this dish, you'll find romaine lettuce, broccoli, cucumber, carrot, green peas, and raw beets. This combination alone will provide nearly 1 pound of vegetables and about 8 grams of fiber. Each of the salads featured in the recipe section will provide 1 pound of vegetables; I hope you enjoy them all and I encourage you to make them your own, too—don't be afraid to mix in different veggie combinations.

Eat a daily minimum of 1/2 pound of raw fruit, above pH 5

Fruits are an essential part of a healthy diet. Just as vegetables provide unique vitamins and minerals, fruits do the same. Plus, fruits are hydrating, are low in calories, and provide plenty of fiber (especially whole fruits eaten with the peel). Approximately one cup of chopped or sliced fruit or one medium-sized piece of handheld fruit is equal to $1/2$ pound and will satisfy your fruit serving for the day. For most handheld fruits, the equivalent will be one medium-sized piece of fruit. Each of the smoothies featured in the Acid Watcher Diet will provide at least $1/2$ pound of fruit. These guidelines are baseline recommendations and do not preclude one from eating more volumes of fruits and vegetables.

When you eat to achieve these goals, you will meet and in some cases even exceed the recommended daily amount of fiber. You won't have to worry about tracking your fiber intake; simply meet the daily fruit and vegetable minimums and you will be covered.

Other foods included in the plan will help increase your fiber intake as well. You'll get to enjoy plenty of nuts and seeds (which complement fruit) and whole grains and legumes that pair well with vegetables. The following table lists a variety of popular foods that are rich in fiber that are excellent for people with acid reflux disease. Though berries have a lot of fiber, they are also acidic. However, as you'll soon see in part III of the book, their acidity can be neutralized or lessened by mixing them with certain alkaline foods.

Vegetables	Grains	Fruit	Nuts/Seeds	Legumes/ Beans
Broccoli	Brown rice	Apples	Almonds	Lentils
Brussels sprouts	Oat and wheat bran	Berries	Walnuts	Chickpeas
Beets	Whole-grain breads	Banana	Flaxseed	Lima beans
Asparagus	Buckwheat	Avocados	Sunflower seeds	Peas
Potatoes	Barley	Pears	Pecans	
Carrots	Rye			
Cucumbers				
Seaweed				
All green leafy vegetables				

You can see that the focus is on food-based sources of dietary fiber—engineered sources such as Metamucil and cardboard-tasting granola bars don't make the cut for two important reasons. First, my goal is to encourage you to shift away from processed foods filled with chemical additives and acidic preservatives, which includes most foods that you might buy in a box, bottle, or package. Buying food instead from the produce section and the bulk bins, where you'll find most grains, seeds, and legumes (often at a cheaper price), is the most direct way to get more whole, fiber-rich foods into your diet.

The other reason is the "natural package of nutrients" that I mentioned earlier in the chapter, which automatically comes with foods high in fiber—it's like getting nutritionally super-sized foods without even asking. Importantly, the vitamins, minerals, and nutrients you'll get when you eat more whole, fresh foods have not been pumped into them in a factory or lab but instead occur organically. You simply cannot replicate this complete package in a supplement, no matter how hard you try. As you work to increase your fiber intake on the Acid Watcher Diet, always think fruits and vegetables first.

CHAPTER 7

Developing Your pH Savvy

THE TRUTH ABOUT ACID/ALKALINE BALANCE AND "HEALTHY" FOODS THAT PEOPLE WITH ACID REFLUX SHOULD AVOID

One important thing about micronutrients, which you get from plant-based and animal-based sources (especially animals that eat a lot of plants), is that they play a role in maintaining a perfect pH balance in your body. That doesn't mean that what you eat will directly affect your balance—in fact, that's one of the more prevailing myths about pH that I will discuss in this chapter—but making sure your diet is balanced will ensure that your body is always getting the tune-up that it needs. As an Acid Watcher, you can establish the best possible diet by using pH correctly—not to maintain your body's pH balance throughout, but to control the amount of naturally and industrially produced low-pH foods that inflame the organs in your aerodigestive tract. To do so is not difficult; in fact, it will be a matter of habit within days. But you do need to acquire just a bit of pH savvy.

Getting to Know pH Better

As you already know, pH is the standard measurement for acidity in the foods you consume. It's important to understand the more nuanced impact of pH on your bodily organs, fluids, and functions. The pH level of the foods you consume will affect your body in some ways but not in others. There are some bodily functions that you cannot control by manipulating your diet. For example, the pH level of human blood in a relatively healthy body always falls within the narrow range of 7.35 to 7.45. It is kept in check by your kidneys, which excrete excess acid through your urine, and by your lungs, which excrete carbon dioxide (a by-product of oxygenation) through the process of exhalation.

Although a life-sustaining pH level in the blood is maintained by this reliable mechanism, the pH levels throughout your body vary from organ to organ, each with its own ideal pH level, depending on the function it performs. For example, the pH of skin is around 5.5, which is slightly acidic, to help defend against pathogenic bacteria. The pH level of saliva, however, is more on the alkaline side, ranging from 6.5 to 7.5. This may allow acidic foods in your mouth to be somewhat alkalized (or balanced) and can even prevent your tooth enamel from corroding when exposed to acidic components in the food you chew. In your stomach, the normal pH is highly acidic, measuring between 1.0 and 4.0, which allows your food to be broken down or digested. Without this process, nutrients from food couldn't be absorbed into your body.

Unlike pH blood levels, the pH levels throughout the body are influenced by the food we ingest, as well as our lifestyle and habits. This includes what we eat or drink, if we smoke or take drugs, and our daily stress level, as well as our exercise and sleeping habits. When these levels fall out of their optimal range, our health can become compromised.

While we can't measure the pH levels of individual organs by taking a urine or blood test—nor do we need to—we can control our exposure to acid through smart diet choices and practice of healthful habits. The ultimate goal should be to allow for acid-damaged tissue to be repaired, and, in the long run, help stall or reduce oxidative stress. This practice of dietary acid management will usher in a range of health benefits—among them reduction of scale-busting cravings and chances for developing chronic disease. We can use the pH scale to our advantage by giving our body the fuel and nutrients it needs to function optimally, and by staying away from additives, harmful chemicals, and select items whose natural acidity can't be neutralized. But first you need to develop the right kind of awareness. Or, if you are an Acid Watcher, we can call it AWareness.

Putting an End to pH Myths

Outside scientific and medical circles, the understanding of the relationship between your body's pH, your diet, your weight, and your health is woefully distorted. Part of the confusion comes from the use of the word *acid* itself. Acid-base balance is not the same thing as gastric acid or dietary acid balance, even though they are all measured on a pH scale. (The role of pepsin is crucial to the distinction between dietary acid and acid-base balance.) Unfortunately, this crude interpretation and application of pH has given rise to a slew of nutritional programs that promote variations of "alkaline" diets, which may have some generic benefits for some consumers but not for people with acid reflux disease.

If you've ever tried an alkaline or pH-balancing diet, you're one of the likely millions of people with acid reflux to have done so. These dietary programs promise to combat an acidic environment by helping restore your pH, or acid-base balance, by curtailing "acidic" foods (measuring below pH 7) that cause a dietary acid overload. The benefits of following this type of diet are said to be numerous and include fat loss, increased energy, and a decreased susceptibility to a range of chronic diseases.

Many pH-centered weight-loss programs also claim that an alkaline diet program can help restore your blood pH balance. This is a biological impossibility. You cannot change or "balance" your blood pH through dietary measures. Your blood pH is maintained through a self-regulating mechanism that relies on communication between the body's acid "buffers"—your blood, kidneys, and lungs. In a generally healthy body, the balance between acid and alkaline in the blood is reliably maintained, irrespective of your diet. You also cannot measure your blood pH with litmus strips, urine tests, or any other type of at-home kit, as plenty of alkaline diets claim. Your urine—which some programs ask you to test periodically—may reflect the acidic components of foods you've consumed earlier in the day, but it will not say anything reliable about acid damage happening in any other part of your body, especially in your gastrointestinal or respiratory organs where this damage needs most urgent repair.

Another major misconception promoted by alkaline diet nutritionists and dieticians is that eliminating "acidic" macronutrients like animal proteins will reduce your acidic overload and make you healthier. Your body is more complex than that and it doesn't always respond to nutrient deprivation the way you'd think. And if you have acid reflux, nutrient depletion is the last thing you should want.

Understanding these two important takeaways will help establish you as an enlightened Acid Watcher. You won't waste time (or money) trying to test your pH because you know that low-acid eating is about reducing tissue damage and inflammation, not about manipulating your blood or urine pH. You also won't be eliminating valuable macronutrients that can aid, even accelerate, your healing from long-term acid exposure.

The pH and Micronutrient Connection

Thanks to the increasing levels of carbon dioxide emission since the industrial revolution a century and a half ago, the pH of our oceans has dropped from 8.2 to 8.1. By inference, you can conclude that the seafood that comes out of the oceans today (even though the commercial seafood we consume is mostly of a farmed variety) is more acidic, and therefore possesses a diminished micronutrient profile, than the seafood that emerged from the oceans before the industrial revolution. Still, even though wild fish caught today is probably less alkaline than the fish in the days of yore, it still offers a range of health benefits not just for Acid Watchers but people in general. In the United States especially, fish is not consumed in the amounts it is in the Mediterranean region and other parts of the world, with most of our dollars going toward red meat and poultry as the animal protein of choice. As an Acid Watcher you should develop AWareness about the varieties of fresh fish in your local markets and grocery stores.

THE ACID WATCHER'S GUIDE TO
EVALUATING DIET FACTS AND TRENDS

Of course, there are other dietary rumors that are more true than false and have even withstood the test of time and scientific scrutiny. For example, a Mediterranean-style diet can really be as good for you as they say it is (with some modifications made for people with acid reflux; more on this to come). This popular way of eating reflects the dietary patterns of several countries in the Mediterranean basin—Spain, France, Italy, Greece, and parts of the Middle East. Typically, the diet is characterized by a high intake of extra virgin olive oil, nuts, locally grown and seasonal fruits, vegetables, legumes, and whole-grain cereals; a moderate intake of fish, poultry, and nonfat dairy products; and a low intake of red meat, processed meats, sweets, and industrially produced baked products. Wine, usually red, is regularly consumed with meals. Adherence to such a diet increases the intake of antioxidants and unsaturated lipids, particularly monounsaturated fatty acids, which have shown positive correlations with longevity and systemic health. Anecdotal evidence of miraculous cancer cures and impossibly long life spans of inhabitants in remote Mediterranean outposts abound and are often attributed to these dietary patterns.

There is also plenty of concrete scientific evidence that the Mediterranean-style diet protects against low-grade inflammation that promotes cardiovascular disease, obesity, and insulin resistance, a precursor to type 2 diabetes. And not only does it help prevent symptoms of these diseases from developing, it has been shown to produce therapeutic effects on these conditions. It's a testament to the truism that it is never too late to change dietary habits in order to improve cardiovascular health. One study showed that a Mediterranean diet had positive effects after just three months of adherence in individuals age fifty-five to eighty! While the evidence on the correlation between the Mediterranean diet and cancer prevention is harder to find, we do know that high red meat and processed meat intake is associated with a higher risk of colorectal cancer, and the adherents to the Mediterranean diet are at lower risk for this disease as well as diabetes and hypertension. The dairy products in the diet may also play a protective role.

Another inspiring diet is DASH (Dietary Approaches to Stop Hypertension). Developed in the 1990s with the purpose of reducing cardiovascular disease, DASH gained a following for not just reducing symptoms of the disease but for the weight loss that accompanied it. The difference between the Mediterranean diet and DASH is that the latter encourages a higher consumption of heart-healthy fats—the kind present in products rich in omega-3 and omega-6—and vitamin D supplements. The Mediterranean diet, in contrast, is naturally rich in vitamin D, as sun exposure tends to be longer in the Mediterranean region than in noncoastal areas. So no supplements are needed there.

The nod to these diets is imbedded in one of the Acid Watcher principles: the requirement that you consume 1 pound of vegetables and 1/2 pound of fruit each day. People have been doing this in Mediterranean cultures for generations, and with DASH since the early 1990s, and we know that it works.

THE BIG BUT ...

However, for an Acid Watcher to embrace this diet without awareness of some caveats would be more detrimental than helpful. The reason is that the Mediterranean-style diet features as some of its staples nutritious but high-acid ingredients that must be avoided. These include wine, tomatoes, vinegar, lemon, and two digestive disruptors, onion and garlic. Of these, wine is the most detrimental to people with acid reflux (although I do offer the options of agave-based liquors [tequila] and potato- or corn-based spirits [vodka] as occasional indulgences in the Maintenance Phase of the diet).

The absence of tomatoes, onions, garlic, vinegar, and citrus foods from the Healing Phase is essential for the acid-damaged esophageal and throat tissue to be healed. But take heart; in this phase, the tastes of garlic, vinegar, and citrus can be substituted in your dishes with spices like sumac, asafetida, dried herbs like savory, and the Acid Watcher go-to condiment Bragg Liquid Aminos. And I do allow modifications for tomatoes, onions, and garlic in the Maintenance Phase. The acidity of tomato can be neutralized by a seedless cucumber; onions and garlic cooked on high heat can be consumed if they are not your trigger foods.

The good news is that I've retained some of the more valuable principles of the Mediterranean-style diet in the Acid Watcher Diet. It is naturally anti-inflammatory, which increases the chances of holding back the free radicals; high in fiber, to keep you satiated and help you lose weight; and high in antioxidants, which will help you fight free radicals. The Acid Watcher Diet has an edge over the Mediterranean-style diet because it is low in dietary acid (natural and chemical), which, as we have seen, is a source of chronic inflammation throughout the body and especially in the aerodigestive tract.

Processed Food Can Ruin the Healthiest Diet: A Takeaway from the Nicotera Study

Back in the 1960s, scientists set out to explore and compare the benefits of the Mediterranean diet on cardiovascular health in a seminal effort that became known as the Seven Countries Study. Because countries bordering the Mediterranean Sea are not identical in their cultural, economic, or even dietary predilections, scientists chose four different cohorts in the region: Crete and Corfu in Greece, Dalmatia in Croatia, and Montegiorgio in central Italy. All the locations represented subtle variations in the diet: the Greek diet had the highest content of olive oil and was high in fruit, the Dalmatian diet was highest in fish, and the Italian diet was high in vegetables. It turned out that the timing of the Seven Countries Study was prescient, as the region was enjoying a period of recovery from the devastation of World War II, but it was still free from the intrusion of the high-fat, high-sugar, highly processed Western diet that spread throughout the industrialized world starting in the 1970s. At the time, the findings in the Seven Countries Study were still being used to evaluate diets in other European countries in an effort to better understand the relationship between diet and cardiovascular disease.

But the truly interesting revelation didn't come until 1996, when researchers returned to the sleepy town of Nicotera in the

Montegiorgio region of Italy, one of the locations in the original Seven Countries Study. While the results from the original study showed that the population of Nicotera exhibited some of the positive effects of the Mediterranean diet—including relatively low incidence of cardiovascular disease—the study conducted in 1996 produced more alarming results. It seemed that the Nicotera residents were showing an increased incidence of cardiovascular disease, cancer, and other inflammatory diseases. They were thus exhibiting the same rising patterns of chronic disease observed in other countries in Europe and around the world.

What did the scientists conclude was the factor for this drastic change over three decades in Nicotera? A deviation from the standard Mediterranean diet that unfolded over the course of thirty-five years, with an increase in consumption of processed, baked, and sugary goods. But the study didn't end there. Some residents agreed to return to the original Mediterranean-style diet and after six months, the news was predictably encouraging. After an extended adherence to the diet, the subjects showed decreased body weight, body mass index, waist circumference, waist-to-hip-circumference ratio, and total body fat.

It seems that one dietary trend can go a long way—backward or forward.

One Last Word About Citrus and Vinegar

You may be surprised to discover that vinegar and citrus are an Acid Watcher's nemeses. If you have experienced acid reflux with some regularity, you have probably heard or read a suggestion that involved a splash of apple cider vinegar or a squeeze of lemon as a relief measure. My patients, often confused about what to eat and what not to eat, ask me, almost daily, questions like "Should I drink apple cider vinegar for my reflux? I heard it's a natural cure," or, "Is it true that lemon juice can heal heartburn?"

These questions have come about as a result of an unproven hypothesis that gained traction over half a century ago: the misguided "alkaline ash" theory. The alkaline ash hypothesis (and its opposite, the acid ash hypothesis) posits that food, after being digested, leaves either an acidic or alkaline residue in the body based on its mineral composition. For example, it's said that lemon leaves an alkaline residue after it is digested, and therefore it's good for the alkalization of the body. As an example of acid ash, it has been proposed that protein and grain foods leave acidic residue that can cause the leaching of calcium from the bones. Provocative as these theories may be, they are yet to be scientifically validated as a means for regulating the body's pH or as a cure for any ailment at all.

For people with acid reflux, the alkaline ash theory is particularly counterproductive because it fails to consider the possibility that food itself, and not its residue, can damage the throat and esophagus. For example, drinking lemon water is widely touted as a good home remedy for people with heartburn—or even just for people who want to kick-start their day. However, the latest research shows that as soon as you drink lemon water, pepsin receptors in the throat are activated. Pepsin, as you have learned, is the enzyme typically located in the stomach whose primary function is to break down protein. It has two forms—active and inactive. When it is inactive, pepsin is basically "asleep" in the stomach. It is activated, or awakened, when it is exposed to acid—such as lemon water or apple cider vinegar. It then goes about doing its job, digesting the food in your stomach as if it were after a meal.

Because pepsin is a floater, people with acid reflux have been shown to have pepsin receptors as far away from the stomach as the esophagus, vocal cords, windpipe, lungs, sinuses, and even the middle ear! So when a small amount of stomach acid reaches the throat, pepsin molecules travel along with it and become attached to the throat and esophagus. The pepsin can then stay in the throat for an extremely long period of time, going in and out of its "sleep mode." Every time you drink that lemon juice, soda, or apple cider vinegar, pepsin "awakens" and starts eating away at the delicate throat tissues as well as the esophageal lining, severely inflaming these organs. The effect is similar to pouring acid over a wound. The only way to stop this corrosive cycle is to keep pepsin receptors that are outside the stomach inactive. Consuming acidic substances like lemon water or vinegar will activate these molecules and cause inflammation way beyond the stomach.

And while we know that acid-activated pepsin will cause inflammation wherever it is found, there is no proof that the "alkaline ash" from acidic food will produce, upon digestion, something that will in any way be beneficial to your general health. For an Acid Watcher, the abundant misinformation associated with lemon juice and apple cider vinegar as "natural treatments" for acid reflux disease is more than just inaccurate, it's outright dangerous.

Another important fact about pepsin is that it becomes most active in an environment that has a pH level between 1 and 4. And it becomes progressively more *inactive* at pH 5 or greater. A person with acid reflux has to be careful because "tissue-bound" pepsin is reactivated every time it encounters food that has a low pH level. (This is another reason that the alkaline ash diet is not a good choice for people with acid reflux; it ignores how the pH of ingested food affects the pepsin that already exists in the throat and esophagus.) During the Healing Phase of the Acid Watcher Diet, foods will be limited to a pH of 5 and above, which will thoroughly quell pepsin activity and allow the esophageal and throat tissues to heal. In the Maintenance Phase, you will be allowed to eat foods measuring down to pH 4, opening up a bigger choice of dietary options.

CHAPTER 8

Breaking Acid-Generating Habits and Establishing Acid-Reduction Practices

Becoming pH savvy is essential for acid reduction, weight management, and long-term health. Devising a customized strategy for stress reduction, sleep improvement, and exercise is another key step. For Acid Watchers, getting rid of habits and practices that exacerbate disease-causing inflammation—such as smoking, drinking certain types of beverages, and eating heavy meals late in the evening is also a crucial task.

If you have acid damage, I can bet that some of your habits have exacerbated your condition. In this chapter, I will explore the most common habits and mistakes that must be broken for the healing to begin, and the positive practices that will help maintain the progress that you will be making.

The Perfect Storm—Kira's Story

I see many patients who are singers, actors, and other professionals for whom vocal cords are not just a vital body organ but a highly refined instrument critical to their livelihood. Singers are especially attuned to changes in their voice and sensitive to any discomfort—whether it is hoarseness, shortness of breath, or obstruction in their throats—they experience during rehearsals or performance. This is one of the reasons they feel acid damage in the upper respiratory tract more acutely than others and are especially eager to find and eliminate the source of their troubles.

Kira was one such patient. At twenty-two, she was a student at a liberal arts college majoring in musical theater. She had noticed, during auditions, that her voice was weaker and she could no longer sustain the high register. She complained about frequent throat clearing and thick mucus in her throat, especially in the morning. She didn't, however, experience any difficulty swallowing or abdominal pain. She tested negative for allergies. A larynx examination revealed the problem: two asymmetric bumps at the vocal folds surrounded by swelling and redness. The bumps and the swelling prevented the folds from closing completely, allowing the air above and below the swelling to escape. This diminished the power of vibrations that Kira needed to deliver the sound she was seeking.

Kira's description of her diet and daily routines provided some clues about the possible origin of the condition. In the mornings, she tended to jump-start her days with diet cola and a bagel with cream cheese. While she didn't drink any tea or coffee, Kira regularly consumed two to three diet colas per day, enjoyed occasional chocolate, and frequently popped breath mints into her mouth. On weekends she relaxed with alcohol—primarily wine and beer. I recognized other telltale signs of dietary acid overload—Kira's daily lunch salad was loaded with tomatoes, onions, or garlic and flavored with vinegar-based dressing. In the evenings, Kira worked at a restaurant. She ate dinner after work, always late at night, right before coming home and crashing in bed after a long day's work. On the evenings Kira didn't work at the restaurant she was busy rehearsing or performing. When she performed on stage, Kira eased her performance anxiety with an occasional joint. After the gig, she grabbed a late-night dinner of pizza or Chinese food on her way home.

While none of these eating or lifestyle habits may seem overtly hazardous to one's health, they produced a bad cumulative effect. Eating dinner late and going to bed shortly thereafter sets the ground for one kind of dietary acid overload. Remember that the stomach requires three to four hours to complete digestion. If you lie down within that time period, the force of gravity will take its course, predisposing partially digested contents in your stomach, coated and infused with gastric acid, to reflux up into the esophagus and the throat instead of down into the small intestine where they belong. Kira's occasional joint smoking and inhaling vapor to reduce stress might have relaxed her, but she didn't do many favors for her delicate vocal cords. Any smoke inhaled is extremely inflammatory to the vocal folds, throat, lungs, and esophagus, where the pepsin is latched onto the tissue, waiting patiently to be awakened.

In the mornings, Kira added fuel to the fire by drinking caffeinated, carbonated soda, which loosened her LES on the lower end of the gastrointestinal tract, while activating pepsin positioned in her upper respiratory tract. It was the perfect storm for an acid overload, and even though Kira was otherwise a healthy young woman, it had derailed the quality of her performance and set the groundwork for more problems to come.

Quit Smoking (All Smoking)

If you haven't lived in a cave or in outer space for the last fifty years, you already know that smoking is a deadly habit. You probably don't need me to reiterate here the destructive path that cigarette smoke blazes through your body. Its connection to chronic and deadly diseases, including cancer, is well documented in science, medical, and popular literature. Its impact on everything from your loved ones (secondhand smoke has been proven to affect innocent nonsmoking bystanders, especially children who are prone to asthma) to your appearance and vitality (smoking accelerates the aging process) is pervasive and insidious.

For Acid Watchers, smoking is an absolute, non-negotiable restriction. Here is a brief statistic to give you a sense of how direct the link is between cigarette smoke and acid damage: 100 percent of smokers have acid reflux disease. In other words, if you smoke, you are guaranteed to develop acid reflux disease throughout the length of your aerodigestive tract—from the pharynx in your throat to the lower esophageal sphincter that holds back gastric acid from entering your esophagus from the stomach. Cigarette smoking is an established risk factor for esophageal adenocarcinoma (cancer of the lower esophagus), esophageal squamous cell carcinoma (cancer of the middle and upper regions of the esophagus), and esophagogastric junctional carcinoma (cancer of the lower esophageal junction, the tissue beneath the LES that separates the stomach from the esophagus).

The physiological damage to these organs from smoke and nicotine present in cigarettes, made even worse if consumed in conjunction with alcohol, is brought on by chemical as well as mechanical changes. We know that nicotine adversely affects the esophageal mucosa by producing free radicals, which leads to oxidative stress injury. Cigarette smoke may also have similar effects on the pharyngeal mucosa, which affects the organ's sensory endings. This could explain why cigarette smokers are more likely to have a relaxed upper esophageal sphincter, which allows mucus from the esophagus to flow back into the throat, spilling onto the vocal cords and even into the lungs. This creates classic conditions for throatburn and its attendant symptoms—swelling of the vocal cords, aspiration (choking sensation), hoarseness, and cough.

Cigarette smoke and nicotine can also predispose smokers to GERD by delaying gastric emptying, decreasing the pressure of the lower esophageal sphincter and thereby allowing gastric acid to backflow into the esophagus and impair its acid clearance mechanism. Smokers are therefore more likely to have both throatburn *and* heartburn.

Another kind of smoke is toxic to people with acid damage, and it comes from the *Cannabis sativa* plant, otherwise known as marijuana. As an Acid Watcher and a doctor I am concerned about marijuana's potential role in the rising rates of esophageal cancer, especially because we are in new and uncharted waters with respect to this popular recreational drug. There is no doubt that fewer Americans smoke marijuana than cigarettes—some 18 million Americans use marijuana compared to 42.1 million who smoke cigarettes, and, according to the *New England Journal of Medicine,* marijuana smokers consume less of their respective product than cigarette smokers do. But while cigarette smoking has overall declined since the 1970s, access to marijuana is likely to increase in the decades to come. The movement to legalize the drug for medicinal and recreational purposes has made great strides between 1996 and 2014, with twenty-three states legalizing marijuana use in some form. And it isn't just gaining general public support; a recent poll of medical professionals revealed that 76 percent supported the use of medical marijuana, as opposed to 54 percent of Americans who support its legalization.

For an Acid Watcher, marijuana can never be considered medicinal. In fact, carcinogenic properties in marijuana are more potent than those in tobacco cigarettes, causing an inflammatory effect on the entire aerodigestive tract—mouth, tongue, vocal cords, lungs, esophagus, and even the bladder. Animal studies also show that marijuana use accelerates growth of abnormal cells. A single joint has four times as much tar as a single cigarette, which may explain why marijuana that is inhaled with less frequency than cigarette smoke can still produce the same long-term effect.

The plant's components activate specific receptors *both* in the brain and in the gastrointestinal region and essentially play off each other. Once stimulated, the receptors in the brain not only help produce the high one experiences but also relax the reflexes that protect us from aspiration and acid regurgitation. Receptors in the mammalian brain that produce pleasure can also influence the regulation of feeding behavior, producing food cravings that marijuana users will recognize as "the munchies." Therefore, marijuana indirectly promotes the deposition of energy as fat into adipose tissues. And we know how weight gain, especially around the waist, promotes GERD and a range of other metabolic problems.

Eliminate Wine, Especially White Wine (pH 3.3), Which Is Even More Acidic Than Red Wine (pH 3.5), and Limit Other Alcohol Intake

This is a tough one. We've heard so much about the health benefits of wine, especially of red wine, with its offerings of antioxidants, cardiovascular disease repellents, and epicurean delight enhancements that make it one of life's greatest pleasures (at least for some). This coveted staple of Mediterranean and haute cuisine is every gourmand's tonic of choice, but unfortunately, it is devastating for people with acid reflux.

With a pH ranging from 2.9 to 3.9, wine is off limits during the Healing and Maintenance Phases of the Acid Watcher Diet. Other alcohol consumption should also be treated with care. In the Maintenance Phase of the diet, a limited amount of agave (tequila), potato-based vodka (including, but not limited to, Chopin, Spud, and LiV) or corn-based vodka (including, but not limited to, Tito's and Balls) is allowed in moderation, but keep in mind that alcohol stimulates gastrin—a hormone that triggers the production of gastric acid—and acid secretion in the stomach. Just like it slows down your reflexes and loosens your tongue, alcohol also delays gastric acid emptying in your digestive tract. It relaxes the lower esophageal sphincter, allowing the acid to travel into places where it doesn't belong. Your esophageal muscle's reflexes become as wobbly as your steps, compromising its ability to clear out the acid with the help of the acid-neutralizing saliva. Studies have also shown that alcohol acutely slows down esophageal movement, or motility. So not only will alcohol relax the LES, but it will also impair motion of the esophagus, thereby making the esophagus a sitting duck for esophageal injury.

Worse, if you smoke *and* drink, studies have shown that concurrent use of tobacco and alcohol may have an additive deleterious effect on the aerodigestive reflexes. So if you smoke and drink, you will exacerbate your acid reflux symptoms exponentially.

Reduce Caffeine Products (Coffee, Tea, Chocolate) and Eliminate Carbonated Drinks (Including the Low-Sugar or Diet Varieties)

If you begin each morning with a cup of coffee, I'm sure this restriction is already making you cringe. And if you've been enjoying six cups of coffee per day since the Nixon administration, you are probably panicking. Just take a deep breath. I don't expect this habit to be broken overnight. It will likely be easier to first reduce the amount of coffee you consume. The good news is that coffee withdrawal symptoms, while unpleasant, will pass in a matter of days, and once they do you'll find that you'll enjoy more energy than when you had to rely on caffeine to start your day.

Coffee is omitted during the Healing Phase of the Acid Watcher Diet for good reasons:

- First, coffee contains the buzz-bringing caffeine, which contains methalxanthine, a chemical also present in tea, sugary and diet soda beverages, chocolate, and many prescription drugs. Methalxanthine has been shown to contribute to a loosening of the LES.

- The second and perhaps more important reason for an Acid Watcher to abstain from caffeine is that it stimulates gastric acid secretion. By imbibing it you are not only awakening the pepsin receptors as the caffeine-infused beverage goes down your esophagus, you are increasing your chances of a greater acid injury in instances of reflux from the stomach, as the undigested content will be further acidified. You need to be caffeine free during the healing stage of the Acid Watcher Diet so the damaged tissue can be repaired. The coffee restriction applies to the decaffeinated variety as well because decaffeinated beverages are never fully caffeine free. You can, however, look forward to the reintroduction of coffee and tea in limited amounts during the Maintenance Phase.

I am less flexible with the carbonated-beverages restriction. All carbonated beverages, whether they are sugary sodas (which are made especially toxic by both the acidity and the insulin-disruptive properties of the added high-fructose corn syrup) or the sugar- and caffeine-free variety, must be eliminated. With or without the presence of caffeine, sugar, or sugar substitutes, the process of carbonation does two things: First, it slightly reduces the pH of any beverage, thereby making it a more acidic and aggressive pepsin stimulant. Your entire gastrointestinal tract feels the pain and the inflammation surge with every sip you take. Second, the gas bubbles in carbonated beverages distend the stomach almost two to one over noncarbonated beverages. Think about stomach distention as a balloon being blown up, its contents shooting up into the adjacent esophagus. Sugary and diet sodas are so corrosive to the delicate tissues of your esophagus and beyond, including the delicate vocal cords, that I liken these substances to the battery acid in your car.

Stop Relying on Processed Foods

Recall from chapter 2 that the primary reason for the dramatic shift from one type of esophageal cancer (esophageal squamous cell carcinoma, or cancer of the upper esophagus) to another (esophageal adenocarcinoma, which affects the lower esophagus) is a result of the radical change in the American or so-called Western diet since the 1970s. This change is categorized by the proliferation and instant availability of large quantities of highly processed, very acidic, extremely addictive, unhealthy foods such as prepackaged meals, salty fatty snacks, sugary sodas, and coffee, which have all become a part of our daily lives, though perhaps not in equal measure. Processed foods are packed with the axis of dietary evil—salt, sugar, and bad fat—and sometimes they are masked so well you can't even taste them. The shift to low-fat, low-sugar, and low-calorie options made matters—and obesity statistics—even worse. Now the products were processed even further, their pH value lowered and the acid quotient heightened.

As these ominous food trends were being promoted and espoused, the pushback started almost as soon as the trend began, with the whole-foods culinary movement. It originated in California, where the legendary chef and restaurateur Alice Waters advocated for a return to plant-based, high-nutrient, natural, local, and environmentally friendly sources of food as the foundation of a healthy and satisfying diet. The movement grew—though not fast enough for people with acid reflux—and was supported by journalists, nutrition experts, physicians, and food writers like Michael Pollan, Mark Bittman, Michael Moss, pediatric endocrinologist Dr. Robert Lustig, and chef and educator Anne Cooper. It took a while, but this agenda is slowly becoming mainstream.

There are promising indications that millennials, a generation born from 1980 to 2000 in the United States, are partaking in the whole-foods movement and rejecting the processed, commercialized, and harmful chemical-laden foods that the previous generations embraced and upon which they grew so dangerously reliant. This is a promising trend for young people, who have made a return to natural, unprocessed foods part of their lifestyle.

Unfortunately millennials have not completely escaped the detrimental impact of dietary acid. In the past year alone, I have diagnosed Barrett's esophagus in nine men and women under age thirty. Even ten years ago this would have been a remarkable clinical finding. And they seemed to be unaware of the relationship between the foods they consume and the condition they are facing—not unlike patients of generations past. But just as bad food is part of a problem, good food must be made part of the solution. Consuming the right food can be part of the prevention and cure.

Acid Watchers have to remember that some natural foods have been processed and thus become more dangerous for them. These are vinegar and fruits, vegetables, and animal-source protein that have been subject to pickling, jarring, fermentation, and preserving. Some of these ancient methods of food preparation and preservation have been rediscovered and reinvented by artisanal makers and creative home cooks, and can produce some delicious outcomes. But if you are in the process of acid damage repair, avoid these temptations because they are all pepsin triggers.

Don't Eat for Three Hours Before Going to Bed

My patients who have tried and succeeded on the Acid Watcher Diet report that of all the diet's behavioral and dietary restrictions, this one was the most difficult to fulfill. We have become so used to eating late into the evening as we socialize, unwind in front of a television set or a gadget screen, or soothe our rattled nerves with food, that we can't imagine our evening routines any other way.

The cultural and economic norms that once delineated our work life from our personal life and separated our working hours from our private time have blurred. Increases in part-time and temporary employment and the presence of a vast, globalized online economy have made standard working hours a thing of the past. Set timing for meals, once so predetermined—breakfast in the morning, lunch midday, and dinner in the evening—are now more of an individual choice than a communal experience or expectation. Sometimes a late-night dinner is the only meal of the day we can actually enjoy with our loved ones, and who would want to give that up, even for health's sake?

For an Acid Watcher, however, lying down or reclining immediately after eating is a hazard for obvious reasons. When you are in a reclined position, the force of gravity pivots the digestion in the opposite direction, projecting the contents of your stomach—which have been pumped up with gastric juice—up instead of down. If you have acid reflux in the lower digestive tract, the already compromised LES is even more poised to let the acidified content into the esophagus where it doesn't belong. So you can add heartburn prevention to a list of metabolic reasons why it is better to eat the last meal of the day earlier rather than later in the evening. Remember that your stomach needs three to four hours to empty out, so the sign outside the Acid Watcher dining area should say "Kitchen Closes at 7:30 p.m. Sharp!"

Hard as it is, every Acid Watcher has to try to break the habit of eating late at night. Think of it as step one toward acid damage recovery. Remember that breaking lifestyle and dietary habits will help usher in the establishment of routines and commitments that will enable the Acid Watcher to reverse acid damage and sustain healthy eating and nourishment practices.

Reduce Stress

In the 1950s, the Hungarian-born chemist, endocrinologist, and researcher Hans Selye coined the word *stress* in reference to a range of physiological symptoms experienced by seriously ill patients who were going through a series of adaptation responses to biochemical changes happening in their brain. He borrowed the term from physics to show how the constellation of psychological and physiological events these patients experienced following a trauma was making them sicker. He gave "stress" a more formal medical designation: *general adaptation syndrome*. A master endocrinologist, Selye knew that stress-induced hormonal changes lead to the development of different types of diseases. Working with the hypothesis that stress affects different brain regions, Selye was particularly interested in the relationship between the chemical messengers corticosterone (aka steroid hormones) and dopamine, and how they produce a stress-coping response in patients.

In the decades since Selye launched this fascinating exploration of the medical condition where psychology and physiology intersect, we've learned a lot about the devastating effects of stress on our well-being, and specifically on our digestive health. This area is the one that interests me, because it has so much to do with acid and pepsin production, proliferation, and inflammation in the gastrointestinal region and throughout the body.

You may ask, how does stress, which originates as a chemical reaction in our central nervous system, affect our digestive health? It has to do with our microbiota, a whole ecosphere of microbes (or bacteria) that regulate digestion in the stomach and play a larger role in our overall health.

Microbiota (or the microbiome) are a pool of microbes that inhabit our entire body. The human gut, where most of them live and flourish with a flood of nutrients, is home to about 100 trillion microbes, with the colon being the organ most densely populated by them. Other parts of the body, such as the skin, vagina, and respiratory tract, also host specific families of microbiota. This microbial community regulates some important metabolic and physiological functions in our body, starting with the immune system at the earliest stages of life. The microbiota regulates, through different mechanisms, other important physiological functions related to energy expenditure, satiety, and steady blood sugar levels. The intestinal microbiota are in touch with both immune cells and, most important, our brain.

The relationship between the brain and the stomach is bidirectional, meaning that the changes in the signals of the central nervous system affect the composition of the microbiota, further disrupting the signals emerging from the nervous system. This relationship is referred to as the Brain Gut Axis. There is much left to learn about how this relationship works and how it affects everything from our cognitive development to our immune, endocrine (fat storage signaling), nervous, digestive, and respiratory systems. We do know two things: that misbalance of the intestinal microbial community can be a source of infection, and that alterations in intestinal microbiota have implications on metabolic functions in the gut and the immune system, ultimately leading to the development of a broad array of gastrointestinal diseases, among them GERD, peptic ulcer, and food allergies and intolerance (antigen-related adverse responses). In addition we also know that stress releases more steroid hormones into one's system, and one of the consequences of increased circulating steroid hormone is an increase in gastric acid and pepsin production. For an Acid Watcher, stress is especially detrimental, because it leads to stimulation of acid and pepsin production both from the gut microbiome and from the "steroid effect."

Increased hormone and enzyme secretion is a serious matter. The consequence of higher levels of corticosterone and cortisol as a result of chronic stress go beyond increased acid production. Cortisol is a hunger stimulant, which is why so many people eat when they are stressed. Worse, when you experience chronic stress you are more likely to have trouble falling asleep or staying asleep. Bad quality of sleep can be as bad for you as no sleep at all. When you get an inadequate amount of sleep, you experience an uptake in the amount of ghrelin, also an appetite-stimulating hormone, so you'll eat more when you do wake up. Simultaneously, poor sleep results in the downregulation of leptin, a hormone responsible for the satiety sensation. So not only will you be hungrier because of the increased ghrelin in your blood, your dimmed satiety signal won't bother telling you to shut that refrigerator door because you are so full you can hardly breathe. So you'll just keep eating.

And, in your fatigued and stress-ridden state, you are less likely to engage in healthy fitness activity, which you know you should be doing, but you have a hundred reasons not to.

That's not all. Over the last three decades, advances in technology forced a larger population to move away from manual to sedentary labor, and more specifically at the computer desk (about 25 percent of American workers now work at a computer). When we do sedentary work, we move less and therefore burn fewer calories. Mental-performance stress delivers another blow to the weight-gain equation. Studies have shown that when we perform work that requires mental strain as opposed to physical strain, we tend to excrete more stress hormones such as cortisol that trick us into thinking we are hungry when we are not. We eat more in response, consuming calories that end up being stored as fat. We will get fatter, more likely in the midsection as we age, and the conditions for GERD development will have been set. Sticking to the rules that follow will help you reduce, in the long term, at least some of the stress effects you may be experiencing.

Improve Your Sleep Patterns

Sleep management has become a more urgent issue over the last several decades because many shifts in our external environment—the demands of work, the accelerated pace, and the social pressures related to globalization and modernizing—have all affected how and when we sleep. We know that stress affects the duration and quality of sleep, and we know that sleep curtailment and obesity are related. Reduced sleep upregulates ghrelin, an appetite-stimulating hormone, and downregulates leptin, a hormone responsible for the sensation of satiety. In other words: the less we sleep, the more we want to eat when we are awake, and the less capable our brain chemistry is to stop us from eating more. So one of the solutions in addition to improving our dietary habits is to assess the extent of stress we are experiencing, how it is affecting our sleep and our weight, and how we can work with medical professionals to redress it. If you are subjected to elevated levels of stress, having trouble initiating and sustaining a full night's sleep, and struggling to maintain healthy weight, I urge you to discuss it with your primary physician. These may be interconnected symptoms, and treatment is highly individualized. Usually it involves one or a combination of therapies—behavioral, pharmacological, and exercise.

These are serious medical challenges with links to acid damage that have to be managed concurrently with the dietary plan. But the solutions don't have to be complicated, expensive, or time consuming. Simple routine changes, such as music therapy (listening to relaxing classical music for twenty minutes before bed) or engaging in muscle relaxation (breathing exercises) that you can practice in the privacy of your home have been shown to improve the quality of sleep in individuals experiencing extreme manifestations of stress such as post-traumatic stress disorder. And then there is always the power of exercise to reduce stress, improve the quality of your sleep, and help you lose weight.

Make Exercise Part of Your Life

Exercise can help correct any dysfunctional sleep patterns or habits, which in addition to disrupting metabolic functions can lead to a greater risk for heart disease, high blood pressure, stroke, and type 2 diabetes. In older adults (age sixty and up), insomnia is an established risk factor in developing obesity and chronic disease. Research shows that if you're struggling with getting a good night's sleep, you might take your running shoes out for a spin before you reach for a package of sleep aids. One random study of sixty adults in this age group found that an aerobic exercise program (three one-hour sessions per week for twelve consecutive weeks) improved the quality and quantity of sleep dramatically. For women with generalized anxiety disorder who experienced sleep disturbance, short-term exercise therapy helped improve sleep initiation and duration, producing a measurable improvement in other symptoms of the disorder. Even people with chronic fatigue syndrome, a debilitating disease that is characterized by persistent, medically unexplained fatigue, pain, sleep disturbance, headaches, and impaired concentration and short-term memory, reported feeling less tired after twelve weeks of consistent exercise therapy that included walking, swimming, cycling, and dancing.

Adding a consistent but strategic exercise regimen (described in more detail in chapter 12) to the Acid Watcher Diet will make overall dietary acid management more effective. We know that when it comes to weight loss, exercise and diet are more effective if they are practiced in conjunction with each other than on their own. Studies have also shown that combined dietary weight loss and exercise improve other aspects of health, including psychosocial factors such as stress or depression in larger increments compared with diet or exercise alone. Carrying a lighter load—in weight and on your mind—can only help in your effort to reverse acid damage.

The 28-Day Blueprint for Reducing Acid Damage, Revving Up Metabolism, and Staying Healthy for Life

CHAPTER 9

The Healing Phase
(Days 1 to 28)

Welcome to the Healing Phase of the Acid Watcher Diet. During this four-week program, your body will begin to heal itself from years of acid damage. When acidic, inflammatory foods are removed starting on Day 1, the stage is set for esophageal tissue repair to begin—and this is the first, critical step toward symptom relief.

The good news is you aren't the first to try my 28-day prescription for low-acid eating; thousands have gone before you and experienced life-changing results. Patients who complete this four-week phase report feeling rejuvenated, up to ten pounds lighter, and free of cravings or deprivation. If you move on from the Healing Phase to the Maintenance Phase of the diet and stick to it as a lifestyle commitment, the results are even more impressive. I have a handful of patients who have lost twenty pounds over a six-month period on the Acid Watcher Diet. In addition to ridding themselves of the reflux symptoms, my patients have reported other benefits, such as reduced LDL cholesterol levels and diminished pain and symptoms of autoimmune diseases such as rheumatoid arthritis and psoriasis.

The success of the Healing Phase is based on five core principles of dietary and behavior modifications that will help you eliminate or reduce inflammation and acid-induced tissue damage to the esophagus and upper respiratory tract. This comprehensive approach will allow your body to heal from acid damage, repairing tissue while also promoting gradual weight loss. Your energy level will increase as your metabolism will get revved up. But it will require commitment and scrupulous attention to detail. Still, my patients continue to be astounded by the payoff.

Acid Watcher Diet Principle #1: Eliminate Acid Triggers

The first principle in the Healing Phase is to **eliminate the Dirty Dozen food items:**

1. **Carbonated sodas:** These include the very acidic sugar and diet sodas, club soda, and flavorless sparkling water.

2. **Coffee and tea:** These especially include bottled iced tea, which is full of acidified preservatives.

3. **Citrus fruits:** These include lemon, lime, orange, grapefruit, and pineapple. These are extremely acidic fruits, measuring less than pH 4. I do allow citrus fruits as a flavoring but only when used on raw animal protein, such as in a marinade for fish or chicken.

4. **Tomato:** Although tomato has a large amount of lycopenes, a natural antioxidant, it is acidic and inflammatory for people with acid reflux because it activates and releases tissue-bound pepsin. If you are concerned that giving up tomatoes means giving up a vital source of lycopene, don't worry; other sources of lycopene are allowed in the Healing Phase (see opposite). Besides, to provide lycopene benefits, tomatoes have to be cooked anyway.

5. **Vinegar:** This staple condiment is extremely acidic because of the fermentation process it undergoes, and all varieties—including apple cider—are pepsin activators.

Best Sources for Lycopene

Lycopene is a powerful antioxidant believed to play a role in preventing cancer and heart disease. Red- and rose-colored fruits and vegetables have lycopene, though not all of them are safe for Acid Watchers because of their pepsin-activating properties. Here is a list of items you can indulge in:

1. Guavas

2. Watermelon: Research shows that watermelon has 40 percent more lycopene per cup than raw tomato. So whenever you crave tomatoes in your salad, just replace them with watermelon in both phases of the diet, especially in summer when the fruit is dense with natural sweetness.

3. Papaya

4. Asparagus

5. Purple cabbage

6. Mango

7. Carrots

6. **Wine:** All varieties of alcohol are carminatives (that is, they loosen the LES). In addition, wine is very acidic, measuring from pH 2.9 (white and rosé pH 3.3) to pH 3.9.

7. **Caffeine:** Coffee and tea are off limits during the Healing Phase, but also be aware of other products containing caffeine, such as over-the-counter and prescription medications, alcoholic beverages, and desserts. Wherever it is present, caffeine is an LES loosener and an increaser of acid production by the stomach.

8. **Chocolate:** This high-nutritional-value indulgence is bad for Acid Watchers, especially those with heartburn. It contains

methylxanthine, which loosens the LES and increases hydrochloric acid production by the stomach. The good news is that the Acid Watcher Diet allows carob, a natural chocolate alternative which is just as delicious in homemade desserts.

9. **Alcohol:** As mentioned earlier, alcohol other than wine is also off limits during the Healing Phase because it is a carminative. But because some alcoholic beverages are not as acidic as wine—such as agave (tequila) or potato- and corn-based varieties (vodka)—I allow a limited amount in the Maintenance Phase.

10. **Mint:** This is a powerful carminative and the Acid Watcher restriction applies to the herb itself, its variation as a spice, and flavored chewing gum.

11. **Raw onion:** This is another powerful carminative that loosens the LES, leaving the door open for refluxed acid. It is also a fructan, which means that it causes the intestines to absorb water, thereby causing bloating. During digestion, onion produces gassiness, especially if it is consumed raw. You should stay away from it completely during the Healing Phase. The good news is that onion is reintroduced in the Maintenance Phase, when it is cooked on high heat.

12. **Raw garlic:** Like raw onion, garlic is a carminative and a fructan and is therefore off limits during the two phases of the diet. The same rules that apply to onion apply to garlic as well.

By removing the Dirty Dozen items, and especially the five classic "trigger" foods of caffeine, carbonation, citrus, chocolate, and cocktails (what I refer to as the 5 C's) from your diet, you will create a sort of digestive clean slate. When this happens, you should begin to experience relief from indigestion and most other types of postmeal discomfort.

Acid Watcher Diet Principle #2: Rein In Reflux-Generating Habits

This means eliminate substances and practices that trigger acid reflux:

1. **Eliminate all smoking:** Cigarettes and other sources of inhaled smoke are carcinogens, LES looseners, and gastric acid release stimulants. You can't get rid of acid reflux or heal the damage to your esophageal tissue if you continue smoking.

2. **Drop processed food:** Preservation methods in prepackaged, jarred, processed, and canned foods require the use of chemicals that are inherently acidic or have properties that loosen the LES. I allow three exceptions in the Acid Watcher Diet: canned tuna, chickpeas, and beans. Canned tuna must be water packed and drained before using. Canned chickpeas and beans must be organic and thoroughly washed to eliminate traces of acidified liquids.

3. **Forget fried foods:** You probably already know that this method of cooking is not good for you because it adds bad fats and empty calories into your diet. What you may not know is that deep-frying oxidizes food, contributing to proliferation of free radicals in your body and therefore setting the stage for chronic inflammation. Fried food is also a notorious LES loosener, which is why so many of us feel the regurgitation effect after eating it. There are other satisfying and easy ways to prepare your meals.

4. **Eat on time:** An Acid Watcher should eat frequently but thoughtfully. During both the Healing Phase and the Maintenance Phase, you will eat three meals and two mini-meals per day between 7:00 a.m. and 7:30 p.m. Although the Acid Watcher Diet is not portion controlled, you should not overeat because a stomach that is too full is a source of intra-abdominal pressure that relaxes

the LES. It is crucial that you don't miss meals and that you eat within the suggested time frame, as this will help curtail nighttime reflux—a cruel sleep stealer—and prevent erratic blood sugar levels, which are often the cause of intense cravings. Mini-meals or snacks will play a big part in keeping cravings in check. (I'll give you the pH-friendly itemized food list to choose from.) Be careful which snacks you choose, though; today's processed snack foods, with the word *Snack* thought of as an acronym, could be accurately described as *Specially Nuanced Adulterated Carbs That Kill*.

Use the following time schedule for consistency:

7:00 a.m.–9:00 a.m.	Breakfast
10:00 a.m.–11:00 a.m.	Midmorning mini-meal
12:30 p.m.–2:00 p.m.	Lunch
3:00 p.m.–4:00 p.m.	Midafternoon mini-meal
6:00 p.m.–7:30 p.m.	Dinner

Close your kitchen by 7:30 in the evening, and allow your stomach three hours to digest food before lying down. This will go a long way toward keeping the gastric-acid-infused contents of your stomach from regurgitating into the esophagus.

Acid Watcher Diet Principle #3: Practice the Rule of 5

The Rule of 5 means that you can consume foods with a pH value of 5 and higher. This eliminates most canned and jarred products, as the preservatives and chemicals used to increase grocery shelf life lower the pH value of any food dramatically. Scientific evidence has shown that most substances registering below 5 on the pH scale—and definitely those that dip below 4—are the most powerful activators of pepsin. By eating according to the Rule of 5, you will help suppress pepsin activity, an essential step for complete recovery from acid damage.

The Rule of 5 is more inclusive than it is exclusive. You'll see a broad range of foods in the following list, and it includes plenty of lean proteins, whole grains, fruits and vegetables, condiments, and spices. Because the Acid Watcher Diet is about balance and moderation as opposed to deprivation, it doesn't exclude carbs, fat, or protein. The only target is highly acidic and processed food.

Here is the sampling of foods that measure pH 5 or higher:

Fish: salmon, halibut, tilapia, trout, flounder, branzino, and sole

Poultry: chicken breast, ground turkey, eggs

Vegetables and herbs: spinach, romaine lettuce, arugula, curly kale, bok choy, broccoli, asparagus, celery, cucumbers, zucchini, eggplant, yellow squash, potato, sweet potato, carrots (not baby carrots), beets (fresh or frozen), cremini mushrooms, basil, cilantro, parsley, rosemary, dried thyme, and sage

Raw fruit: banana, Bosc pears, papaya, cantaloupe, honeydew, watermelon, lychee, and avocados

Dried fruit: dates, raisins, shredded coconut

Nuts and seeds: cashews, pecans, pistachios, walnuts, pumpkin seeds, sesame seeds, almonds, pine nuts

Spreads: fresh, raw, organic peanut butter and almond butter

Cheese: Parmesan, mozzarella, feta, and other select hard cheese

Bread and grains: old-fashioned rolled oats, whole-grain pasta, 100% whole-grain bread, whole-grain wheat flour

Sweeteners: agave nectar (a borderline pH value food; see page 129 to learn how to use safely)

Condiments: Celtic salt, olive and coconut oil, Bragg Liquid Aminos, hemp protein, vanilla extract, white miso paste

These are options that provide endless variations for satisfying meals.

Acid Watcher Diet Principle #4: Make Positive Food Choices

The Acid Watcher Diet is popular with patients who are not fond of rigid portion control and calorie counting, and I am one of those. Don't get me wrong; I am not advocating consuming huge meals, which are especially difficult for Acid Watchers to process without reflux. Meals and snacks should be sensible in size, and you will find that over time you will want to eat less because you will be consuming more fiber and spacing out your meals in reasonable intervals to prevent hunger from setting in. Remember that the Acid Watcher Diet provides you with all the macronutrients that your body needs, and when you eat a macronutrient-inclusive diet, you ensure greater appetite satisfaction. You also get to experience other positive side effects such as diminished bloating, a trimmer belly, and more energy. Here's what you have to do to obtain quick results:

1. *Introduce more fiber into your diet.* Fiber is crucial, as it performs the function of a broom that sweeps all the waste from your stomach, aiding in healthy digestion and esophageal protection and delaying digestion. By increasing your fiber intake you can leave the food cravings—and extra pounds—behind. You don't need to rely on supplements to increase your fiber intake.

2. *Eat a daily minimum of 1 pound of vegetables above pH 5, half of which should be consumed raw.* One pound may seem like a lot, but if you enjoy these vegetables throughout the day, you'll find it's easily doable. For example, five medium-sized carrots is approximately 1 pound; consume half of these raw as snacks, and include the rest in a soup or stir-fry later in the day. Four handfuls of string beans is also approximately 1 pound, and 5 cups of spinach is about 1/2 pound. The typical salad one gets at a salad "bar" is often at least 1 pound.

3. *Eat a daily minimum of ¹/₂ pound of raw fruit, above pH 5.* For example, a handful of cubed cantaloupe with a banana is approximately ¹/₂ pound. The fruit in Dr. Aviv's Berry Smoothie Blast (page 158) is also roughly ¹/₂ pound.

4. *Be aware of borderline-pH-value foods that are bad for Acid Watchers.* Reflux-inducing substances may include condiments and natural products that are pH friendly (pH 5 and higher) but should be avoided by people with acid reflux. Among these are items on the Dirty Dozen list in Rule #1—coffee, onions, tomatoes, citrus fruit, vinegar, garlic, mint, and chocolate. But if you have acid reflux, you must also beware of the following items:

> Seed oils
> Peppers
> Berries
> Honey
> Organic agave

Let's look at these separately:

Seed oils such as sunflower, safflower, canola, and sesame are by definition acidic because their extraction process involves the use of chemicals and preservatives. Instead, I recommend using extra virgin olive oil, cold pressed only and unfiltered, if available. These varieties have a higher pH value and taste better. Coconut oil is another option.

Peppers are, by most measures, superfoods, high in pH value and packed with nutrients and antioxidant properties. They are, however, considered acidic because their digestion stimulates production of pepsin. This is the reason I exclude pepper-based spices from the Acid Watcher Diet but allow the introduction of sweet peppers in the Maintenance Phase, if they are consumed cooked, as in grilled, roasted, or sautéed.

What 1 Pound of Vegetables or $^1/_2$ Pound of Fruit Looks Like in the Grocery Cart

Some people get a little alarmed when they hear the 1 pound of vegetables and $^1/_2$ pound of fruit per day rule, but I tell them not to worry; to comply with this rule you don't have to run out to buy a bigger refrigerator or hoard the contents of the entire fruit and vegetable section of your local bodega. Just to give you a sense of how reasonable this requirement is, I've broken down the contents of a sample grocery bag into 1-pound and $^1/_2$-pound increments.

Approximately 1 pound of vegetables is contained in one of the following items:

- 1 English cucumber
- 2 zucchini squash
- 1 small head of cabbage
- 1 bag of spinach (which will reduce to less than a cup when steamed, blanched, or sautéed)
- 1 bundle of asparagus
- 4 celery stalks

Approximately $^1/_2$ pound of fruit is contained in one of the following items:

- 1 banana
- $^1/_4$ of a large papaya, which yields $1^1/_2$ cups of fruit
- $^1/_4$ of a 7-pound baby watermelon, which yields $1^1/_2$ cups of fruit
- 1 pear
- 1 apple (for Maintenance Phase only)
- $^1/_2$ container of strawberries (for Maintenance Phase only!), which yields $1^1/_2$ cups of fruit
- 1 Haitian mango (for Maintenance Phase only!), which yields $^1/_3$ cup of fruit

In short, if you eat a healthy salad and two vegetable sides per day, you will fulfill the vegetable requirement. You can fulfill your daily fruit requirement by eating a few slices of watermelon and a banana. Or, just toss a few raw vegetables and fruit into a blender for a smoothie and call it a day.

Berries are also nutrient-packed and delicious fruit, but they can still produce heartburn from pepsin stimulation. Berries are, however, allowed in both phases of the diet *if* they are balanced by acid neutralizers such as almond milk, non-GMO (genetically modified organism) soy milk, rice milk, and coconut milk. (See page 70.) One way to consume berries safely is through a smoothie, which, in combination with nondairy milk, can be an alkalizing, palate-pleasing combo.

Honey is a natural, anti-inflammatory condiment that stimulates pepsin production. Its pH value is slightly below 5, so it is not allowed in the Healing Phase unless it is in combination with acid neutralizers such as nut butters or raw animal protein (as in a marinade). As long as honey is not your trigger food, feel free to enjoy it in the Maintenance Phase of the Acid Watcher Diet.

Organic agave, another natural sweetener, also falls just a touch short of the Rule of 5. With a pH of 4.3 to 4.8, it is allowed in the Maintenance Phase as a condiment, but in the Healing Phase it is only permitted as a marinade for the more alkaline animal protein. Agave is especially good when paired with miso paste as a marinade for fish or poultry, which is then cooked. Another alkanizing ingredient for agave is nut milk.

5. *Balance your vegetable and protein daily intake.* Practicing positive food choices means placing greater emphasis on vegetable intake. If you eat poultry or fish for lunch, you should consume

a vegetarian dinner. Conversely, a vegetarian lunch should be followed by a poultry or fish dinner. The rationale for eating at least one vegetarian meal a day is that higher consumption of vegetables (as well as fruit) is associated with a lower risk of mortality, particularly cardiovascular mortality. It is also another way to maximize your fiber intake.

6. *Substitute products wisely.*

- Choose grass fed/organic over farmed animal protein.

- Choose a higher omega-3 to omega-6 ratio (seafood).

- Choose organic fruits and vegetables unless they have thick protective skin (for example, banana or watermelon).

- Choose organic peanut butter, preferably freshly ground, as processed, industrially made peanut butter is more acidic.

- Replace processed table salt, which has been depleted of its essential minerals, with Celtic salt.

- Eat 100% whole-grain bread. This includes rye, spelt, wheat, barley, and oat. When the grain has been broken into pieces as part of the bread-making process, all the parts must be used. Some examples are Bread Alone Organic Whole Spelt Bread and Food for Life Ezekiel 4:9 Bread Original Sprouted Organic. All of the bran, germ, and endosperm must be present. If you can't get 100% whole-grain bread, choose one that doesn't have preservatives or artificial flavors.

- The only beverage you should consume during the Healing Phase is water. If you can't stand plain water, you can add a cube of watermelon to make the water slightly sweeter. Alternatively, you can add a few thin slices of cucumber to make the water more savory.

- When eating out, order chicken or seafood that is either steamed, roasted, baked, or grilled—never fried!

Why Celtic Salt Is Better for Acid Watchers Than Regular Table Salt

No doubt you've heard warnings about how bad salt can be for your health, especially if you have cardiovascular disease, high blood pressure, or diabetes. It is tempting to think that such a generic reference to salt encompasses all of its varieties, but that's not the case. Salt, which is a naturally occurring element that contains essential minerals, is far from being bad for you. What is bad—even toxic—is processed table salt. Unfortunately, this is the variety that most people use to flavor their food. Subjected to extremely hot temperature during processing, the crystals of naturally occurring salt undergo an extreme chemical transformation in which they lose nearly all of their nutrients. Instead, they are infused with additives that make the crystals more uniform, long-lasting, and powdery. Like all toxic materials, additives in salt cause an inflammatory response in your body. One such response is water retention.

In contrast to regular table salt, Celtic salt is a naturally harvested whole-crystal sea salt. You know it is natural because it is grayish rather than snow white and the crystals appear in different shapes and sizes. Celtic salt is produced today using the low-tech methods established in Brittany some two thousand years ago. That method allows Celtic salt to retain all of its minerals, electrolytes, and digestive enzymes, which are beneficial rather than damaging to your health.

You'll notice that Celtic salt is less "salty" than the table salt you are probably used to. That's why some of the Acid Watcher recipes call for what seems like excessive amounts of salt. As you get used to flavoring your food with Celtic salt, you'll be able to determine which amount suits you best. Remember that because Celtic salt is so pure, it is going to be a more subtle seasoning.

Acid Watcher Diet Principle #5: Become a Quintuple Threat in the Kitchen

The fifth principle of the Acid Watcher Diet is to learn how to prepare food without hassle. If you can **roast, sauté, grill, poach,** and **blanch,** you can prepare delicious meals with minimal effort. These are straightforward, strategic cooking techniques that should become standard use in your home kitchen (if they aren't already). With just these five cooking methods, you'll be capable of producing a limitless variety of meals. Even if you're a novice cook, you'll find that these techniques are easy to learn and improve upon. Consider yourself experienced in the kitchen? Think of this section as an opportunity for repertoire expansion, or a reminder of techniques you may have overlooked. Every Acid Watcher can benefit.

ROASTING: This cooking method infuses root vegetables and poultry with subtle succulence and richness. The challenge for an Acid Watcher is to come up with alternatives to standby spices, herbs, libations, and citrus (think peppers, garlic, wine, and lemon) that make roasting poultry like turkey and chicken so extraordinary. But I found that using a mix of ground fennel, cumin, coriander, celery seeds, and ginger produces flavors just as exceptional, if not more aromatic. Instead of basting with wine, you can baste with Homemade Chicken Broth (page 229) or a splash of water that will give poultry an attractive and delicious golden crispiness. When you roast a chicken, line the bottom of the pan with parboiled Yukon Gold or sweet potatoes and they'll sop up all the juices and create a comfort food meal to remember.

With root vegetables (carrots, beets, butternut squash, sweet potato), a combination of cinnamon, Celtic salt, cumin, and ginger will provide an exotic-flavored side dish that can be served straight out of the oven, at room temperature, or the next day. These are the important tips to remember: Start at a high temperature (375 to 450°F.) and lower the temperature twice (see individual recipes for time intervals), each time by 25 to 35 degrees. Root vegetables should be roasted on a baking sheet lined with parchment paper and flipped over every twenty minutes until done to prevent burning.

Poultry, if roasted whole, should be trussed and cooked resting on the back, with the breast away from direct flame.

SAUTÉING: It sounds fancy, but if you've ever prepared a hot meal for yourself, your family, and your friends, chances are you've sautéed something. It works especially well for relatively small portions—fillets of fish, chicken breast, or sliced vegetables—that cook quickly on high heat and provide a complete one-dish (or one-skillet) meal in a jiffy. Sautéing is one of my favorite cooking methods for busy people, as most Acid Watchers are. It does not require hours of time spent toiling away in the kitchen but instead can guarantee a satisfying, flavor-packed meal in less than thirty minutes. This technique—like all others—improves with experience, but it is reasonably easy even for a novice to master. You need the following equipment and knowledge:

1. *A nonstick, round sauté pan.* But don't rush out to buy one if you don't already own one. A frying pan or a skillet will do fine, and most kitchens have at least one of those.

2. *Cook, at least initially, on high heat.* I find that controlling temperature is easier on a gas stovetop, but if you have an electric stove, medium-high heat is probably the safest. Heat a teaspoon or two of olive or coconut oil in the pan before you place any fish, chicken, or vegetables in it so the food will brown quickly. Watch for the sizzle, which is evidence that you have enough heat to cook your ingredients properly, but avoid spattering by keeping a safe distance from the pan.

3. *Use a wide, long spatula* (preferably silicone and slotted) to flip fillets (chicken or fish) to prevent scratching the surface of the nonstick pan.

4. *Sauté fish and chicken for the correct amount of time.* Freshwater fish (tilapia, bass, sole, branzino, and flounder) cook quickly, one to two minutes on each side. Chicken breast takes longer; you want it to be fully cooked but not overdone, which makes it dry and stringy. I cook it for two to three minutes on each side, turn off the pan, and cover it completely for another two minutes to make sure the meat is cooked all the way through but has retained its juiciness.

5. *Sautéing time for vegetables varies.* Generally speaking, root and leafy vegetables like carrots, parsnips, fennel, leeks, cabbages, kale, Swiss chard, collards, and radicchio get sweeter and softer the longer you sauté them. Periodically tossing the vegetables will prevent sticking, and adding a sprinkle of water will allow for steaming that makes the texture of the vegetables silkier. More watery vegetables, like zucchini and eggplant, should be flash sautéed (cooked quickly on high heat, for a caramelized, crispy, and flavorful outside and a juicy interior) to retain their crunchiness and prevent them from becoming soggy.

GRILLING: For an Acid Watcher, grilling, especially fish, provides an opportunity to infuse entrée proteins with flavor that might otherwise only come from acidic marinades and spices. I've found that the best natural flavor enhancer is a cedar plank or a cedar wrap, which is available in the fish section of most grocery stores. The smokiness released from the charred cedar plank infuses a fish fillet with an earthy aroma so intense that the only other additional spice you'll need is a dash of Celtic salt. Grilling on a cedar plank or wrap requires only one extra but easy step— soaking it in water for at least fifteen minutes (follow the instructions that accompany grilling planks) before grilling, to prevent burning. This method doesn't change the general rule for grilling fish, which is two to three minutes on each side for medium rare (salmon, tuna), and three to six minutes on each side for well done (halibut, swordfish, and bass).

You can use cedar skewers for grilling shrimp, scallops, and squid to produce tasty dishes that do not rely on acidic flavorings.

POACHING: When it comes to poaching fish, I like to follow the advice of the great American chef and restaurateur Alice Waters, who recommends the method of shallow poaching, in which a fillet of fish (fresh fish or steak) is submerged in flavored water that simmers at the bottom of the pan. White wine and lemon are traditional poaching liquids, but as Acid Watchers, we can't rely on these acidic standards. Instead, I recommend a medley of fresh herbs and aromatics in water—fennel fronds, ginger, dill, parsley, and fresh bay leaf, if available—which infuse foods with fresh, organic flavors. You can also poach fish in Vegetable Stock (page 231). Poaching fish takes three to seven minutes, depending on the thickness of the fillet, and produces a delicate, flaky texture. To add another layer of taste, I recommend serving fish with a sprinkle of fresh dill and toasted sesame seeds.

Poaching fruit is one of the easiest and most satisfying methods to prepare Acid Watcher–style desserts. In the Healing Phase, pears and raisins are a great pairing, and the Maintenance Phase expands the list to include certain varieties of apples and dried fruit. Fresh fruits, such as pears and apples, have to be peeled, cored, and cut in half (pears) or quarters (apples). The poaching liquid can be flavored with cinnamon, vanilla bean, star anise, and cloves. (See page 138 for more details.) In poaching, the fruit (unlike fish) has to be fully submerged in the liquid to cook evenly, and it should retain its shape and a little of its crunch when you take it out to cool. Fresh and dried fruits can be simmered over low heat for up to thirty minutes, covered, and can be left in the liquid to cool. To rev up flavor, remove the fruit with a slotted spoon, bring the poaching liquid to a boil, and reduce by two thirds to make a syrup. Serve cold.

BLANCHING: Some vegetables—especially if they are green—were made for blanching. Asparagus, string beans, broccoli, peas, and Brussels sprouts become a brilliant green after they are blanched, retaining their essence and crunch without adding a single ingredient or calorie. The five-step process couldn't be simpler: just bring a pot of Celtic-salted water to a boil, add the vegetables, cook for five to seven minutes, drain, and place in a bowl of water with ice. The ice bath "shocks" the vegetables by stopping the cooking process, so they don't get soggy. Eat them as is or add them to your salad.

Food as Medicine Is More Than "Eat Your Vegetables"

I am aware that more experienced cooks and food enthusiasts may be looking at these five Acid Watcher Diet rules and wondering how they can hope to make basics like soups, stews, salads, side dishes, and other basic culinary concoctions without the accent that herbs such as garlic and onion allow, or make salad dressings without the tangy accent of vinegar or citrus fruit. Is there hope for a satisfying dessert without chocolate? Well, despair no more, all you epicurean-minded Acid Watchers. I believe that a healthy, low-acid diet can be delicious if you think about your restrictions creatively. When it comes to food, nature has more than one option for you to choose from, and the items I include can be found in your local grocery store, farmers' market, or health food store.

In the Healing Phase of the diet, you can use **fennel** and the Indian spice **asafetida** in place of **onions** and **garlic.** You can use **sumac** in place of lemon and citrus. And try **carob** in place of chocolate. You can make your salad dressing creamier with tofu spread or avocado and replace the tang of citrus (or soy sauce, if you like your salads more Asian style) with **Bragg Liquid Aminos. Star anise** and **cloves** can spice up your desserts.

ASAFETIDA (as-sa-FEH-ti-da): This spice isn't easy to find at your local grocery store, but it is available online (amazon.com and other vendors) as well as in Indian and Persian markets. It's a shame that a spice prized for its medicinal properties—in the ancient world it was used as treatment for maladies ranging from baldness and bronchitis to indigestion and scorpion bites—is so unfamiliar to contemporary eaters. Extracted from a fennel-like plant in the mountains of Afghanistan, this spice traveled southeast through Iran and settled in India, where it continues to be a ubiquitous flavor enhancer for vegetarian dishes. You've probably tasted a hint of asafetida in Worcestershire sauce or Indian-style curries. The spice may not be in demand for ordinary consumers because of its uninviting smell. In fact, *foetida* means "stinking" in Latin, and the spice is often referred to as "the devil's dung." The smell, however offensive it may seem at first, recedes completely in the heat of cooking (especially when combined with olive oil) and acquires a subtle flavor reminiscent of sautéed onions and garlic. For Acid Watchers who can't enjoy onions and garlic but want to experience the depth they bring to all savory dishes, asafetida is a welcome rescue, especially during the Healing Phase of the diet.

FENNEL: You'll find this vegetable—a white bulb with light green stalks and darker green, fragrant fronds—in just about any grocery store, where it is likely to be mislabeled as "anise." Although fennel and anise share a strong licorice scent, fennel is a flowering plant whereas anise is more of a seed (not to be confused with *star anise,* a popular flavoring in cuisines of Asia) that is used as a primary ingredient in absinthe and that you would recognize in French pastis or Greek ouzo. Fennel, however, is a vegetable and an herb, depending on how you want to use it. In Italy—where it continues to be revered as it once was by Greeks and Romans—fennel bulb can be fried, braised, puréed, and consumed raw in salads. Fennel, both the bulb and the fronds, is a natural pairing for any seafood, which is why it is so popular in port cities like Marseilles, France. The entire plant can be used to flavor meat and vegetable stocks and can take the place of onions in soups, salads, and vegetable sautés that call for onions. Fennel is an excellent source of potassium, vitamin C, and fiber; in animal studies, fennel's phytonutrient compound has been shown to reduce inflammation and cell mutation.

SUMAC: A staple in Middle Eastern and Mediterranean cooking, this vibrant, garnet-colored spice is derived from the berries of a subtropical flowering plant native to northern Africa and North America. During antiquity, in the countries of the Levant—Iran, Turkey, Sicily, and northern Africa—sumac added a sprinkle of tartness to stews, meat, fish, and vegetables until the Romans introduced lemon for a fresh tang of sourness that expands the flavors of so many foods. Nowadays, sumac remains popular mostly in professional kitchens but is slowly being discovered by savvy, health-conscious home cooks. Studies have shown that sumac is high in antioxidant properties with benefits for cardiovascular health, glycemic control, and lower cholesterol.

CAROB: A tree pod native to the eastern Mediterranean region and grown in California, carob is technically a member of the legume family. It is a low-fat, caffeine-free, stimulant-free alternative to chocolate that has long been a staple of the vegan diet. Cocoa's health benefits differ from carob's, but one significant nutritional benefit of carob is that it is packed with calcium and pectin, a soluble fiber. It is also the basis for the new Acid Watcher Diet desserts in the Healing Phase, which will satisfy your sweet tooth without compromising the luxurious texture and scents we associate with chocolate desserts. Carob is more broadly available in powder form (great for cakes, frostings, and syrups) and chips (for cookies, bars and trail mixes, and muffins). Like chocolate, carob is a great companion to peanut butter and vanilla, which gives an Acid Watcher a few healthful options for satisfying dessert cravings.

STAR ANISE: Native to China and Vietnam, star anise is the fruit of a tree that, as its name suggests, is star shaped. When dried, it is used as a spice in the kitchen and as a remedy for indigestion and other ailments in homeopathic medicine. It is one of the spices found in the popular Chinese five-spice and Indian garam masala ground mixes. As a whole spice, star anise is used to flavor savory dishes such as slow-cooked Asian soups and stews containing red meat, poultry, and pork. In the Western world it is used more commonly as a dessert flavoring in rice pudding, pies, and fruit compotes. I like to use it when poaching fruit. Its flowery aroma is far more rewarding in taste and health benefits than the artificial, sugary, and citric components that Acid Watchers need to avoid.

CLOVE: The flower of an evergreen tree that grows in the spice islands of Indonesia, clove is a potent, sweet aromatic that can be used in savory dishes (lentils, chili, cold soups) and desserts (pumpkin pie). From a medicinal perspective it is a natural magic bullet: an antiseptic, antioxidant, antiflatulence, and anti-inflammation agent. In short, it is a perfect Acid Watcher spice. But be careful with it in the kitchen—using too much can overwhelm a dish. If using it as a whole spice in a fruit-poaching liquid, limit yourself to two or three flowers. Cloves are also sold in ground form. Like all spices, the pods lose some of their essential oils and nutrients in the grinding process, but when it comes to baking, it's the only way you can use them. I have included clove in several baked dessert recipes in the Maintenance Phase. Just make sure you don't put too much into the mix—no more than $1/4$ teaspoon.

Healing Phase Food List

Dairy (if you are not lactose intolerant or if dairy is not your trigger food)

Blue cheese

Butter (organic)

Hard cheese—Dublin, Parmesan, Asiago, mozzarella, Cheddar

Tree Nuts

Almonds

Walnuts

Cashews

Pistachios

Dairy Alternatives

Almond milk

Soy milk (plain)

Rice milk

Condiments and Spreads

Almond butter

Peanut butter (preferably freshly ground and organic)

Bragg Liquid Aminos (soy sauce alternative)

Spices

Ginger

Sumac

Celery seed

Cumin seed

Fennel seed

Coriander seed

Fish and Seafood

Lobster (boiled)

Shrimp (boiled)

Crab meat

Halibut (poached)

Salmon (grilled)

Octopus (grilled)

Sardines (fresh, if available)

Tuna (in water, canned)

Tuna (seared)

Tilapia

Sole

Branzino

Flounder

Swordfish

Bass

Cod (broiled)

Poultry and Meat

Eggs

Turkey (fresh, roasted)

Chicken (grilled)

Beef (sirloin)

Grains

Multigrain bread (Bread Alone)

Brown rice

Rolled or steel-cut oats

Whole-wheat fusilli

Barley

Buckwheat groats

Ezekiel 4:9 Flax (available at Whole Foods and Trader Joe's)

100% whole-grain bread

Ezekiel 4:9 Sesame

Whole-wheat fiber bread

Legumes

Peas (green)

Peas (black-eyed)

Edamame

Cannellini

Vegetables

Artichoke

Cucumber

Fennel

Radicchio

Eggplant

String beans

Brussels sprouts

Zucchini

Cauliflower

Romaine lettuce

Spinach

Broccoli

Celery

Iceberg lettuce

Swiss chard

Asparagus

Kale

Cabbage

Cucumber

Mushrooms

Russet, Yukon Gold, red, and sweet potato

Beets

Carrots

Herbs

Cilantro

Ginger

Basil

Parsley

Fruits

Avocado

Black olives

Watermelon

Lychee

Butternut squash

Banana

Papaya

Dates (Halawi, Delilah)

Dragon fruit

Honeydew

Pumpkin

Pear

Lemon (only when used on raw animal protein products)

What If Symptoms Persist?

You may find that even when you follow the rules, you still experience occasional digestive issues. If that's the case, some of the items in the preceding list may be your trigger foods. For example, some people with acid reflux have noted difficulty with the digestion of foods such as eggs (especially egg yolks), beans, and dairy (these are common irritants even among those who may not have reflux issues). Eggs contain lysozyme, an enzyme that can wreak digestive havoc for some; beans are high in oligo-saccharides, a complex sugar that can be difficult to digest; and dairy can prove problematic if you can't properly process lactose, the predominant form of sugar found in most foods produced from cow's milk.

The Problem with Cow's Milk

Patients often ask me if they can have dairy in their diet, and I always urge them to be careful. Yes, I allow some dairy products such as certain cheeses in the Healing Phase and yogurt and kefir in the Maintenance Phase because of their probiotic content. But cow's milk is best left to the mammals for whom nature intended it—calves. There is a lot of controversial science on the study of cow's milk, but there is enough evidence to suggest that it is an inflammatory agent. And since the Acid Watcher Diet is an anti-inflammation diet, I am hesitant to recommend it despite the pH value. But if cow's milk is your weakness, you might want to transition out of it by switching to a healthier and delicious goat's milk.

Surprisingly, it is quite common that one person tolerates one type of food very well, yet another person can't tolerate that food at all. Over the years, I've found that some other examples of trigger foods are grapefruit, pineapple, bread, and pasta. Since carminatives as a group can be problematic for people with acid reflux, they'll be omitted altogether from your diet during the Healing Phase. (That's why you don't see radish and raw horseradish on the Healing Phase food list.)

If you continue to experience either traditional heartburn reflux symptoms (heartburn or regurgitation) or throatburn reflux symptoms (chronic cough, hoarseness, constant throat clearing, or a lumplike sensation in the throat) after following the Healing Phase for a minimum of 21 days, you may want to consider keeping a food diary to help identify any of your personal food irritants. Recording what you've eaten over the last day in a food journal will help you see any patterns in your symptoms. You may notice that you experience midmorning reflux only after you've had eggs at breakfast, or the irritation in your throat could appear just on the days on which you've snacked on cheese or had milk with breakfast.

If any of the foods you consume, regardless of their pH level, cause a negative reaction, it's important to remove that type of food. Doing so will end any continuing inflammation that may be disruptive to complete healing and relief from symptoms.

When You Fall off the Wagon

In the years that I've prescribed the Acid Watcher Diet, I have yet to see a patient who hasn't experienced an improvement in at least one of their symptoms after following the 28-day Healing Phase—except when they don't follow the rules. In fact, I've come up with a matrix of questions that can help me predict which symptoms will be alleviated by measuring the extent of the patient's compliance with the individual rules. Over the years, patient feedback has revealed some common challenges in compliance. Here they are, along with some advice on how to manage them.

1. As I already mentioned, behavioral changes are the most difficult to make, so the number one difficulty that my patients have reported with the Healing Phase was giving up their morning coffee. So don't fret if you just can't do it, at least at first. Just try to release your habit gradually by reducing how much you consume.

If you need two cups of coffee in the morning to get going, reduce it to one. If you need one cup, have half a cup instead, etc.

2. The other stubborn habit is eating after dinner. My advice is not to do anything radical like sealing your refrigerator door with crazy glue, setting booby traps all over the kitchen floor, or locking yourself in an attic for the night. Just be aware of your habits. You'll find that if you follow your eating schedule of three meals and two mini-meals and increase your fiber intake, eventually the cravings (and the habit) will subside.

3. Regarding giving up alcohol and wine: I know it's painful. But just do it.

4. Giving up the vinegar in salad dressing seems drastic to my patients at first. I can't tell you how many times I've heard "What is salad dressing without vinegar!?" to which I always reply how simple and delicious it is to dress salad with a mix of olive oil, herbs, and Celtic salt, all of which bring out the natural goodness of fresh vegetables. But if you must feel tartness to enjoy your salad, get the herb mix Savory, which actually tastes like vinegar. Or add sumac to your salt. A mix of carrot and ginger blended with Bragg Liquid Aminos will also satisfy your "sour" tooth. You can also make the dressing creamier with avocado or tofu spread. If you still find yourself in a constant state of salad-driven despair, a little ranch, blue cheese, or Caesar dressing won't kill you. (Especially if you know you are about to go on a garlic bender anyway.)

5. Another Healing Phase challenge is recognizing the "hidden" processed foods—especially cold cereals, which have a lot of preservatives that can loosen the LES, and store-bought granola bars. I found that a cereal habit is easier to kick if you substitute it by having an Acid Watcher–friendly toast and spread, which will be more filling and less sugary. For bars, I always remind patients that Dr. Aviv's Power Bar (page 165), which contains ten almonds, two

dates, and a teaspoon of fresh peanut butter (the processed variety is too acidic), is a delicious medley. Add raisins, dried apricots, and carobs to make the mix more gourmet.

6. The final complaint even before the Healing Phase begins is "How can I eat ANYTHING if I can't have onion and garlic?" I remind patients that their fears will dissipate when they learn to use spices creatively. A combination of ginger, cumin, and cilantro; or oregano, paprika, and salt; or saffron; or asafetida, which is intense and satisfying enough to make the memories of onion and garlic fade away. And when I mention that the fabulous duo of onion and garlic will be back, cooked (if it isn't your trigger food!), in the Maintenance Phase, the office lights up with smiles.

Now Let's Get Cooking!

In the next chapter you will discover dozens of recipes for breakfast, lunch, dinner, and mini-meals during the Healing Phase. You'll also find a two-week sample meal planner designed to take the guesswork out of low-acid eating.

CHAPTER 10

The Healing Phase Meal Planner with Recipes

Getting Started

For Acid Watchers who prefer to follow a diet menu for 28 days without the hassle of planning day-to-day meal sequences, I have designed a very easy-to-follow weekly schedule of meals that you can repeat four consecutive times for the total of 28 days to complete your month of healing. If, however, you would prefer to have more flexibility in meal planning, you can devise your own daily meals from the selections I've organized under Breakfast, Mini-Meals, Lunch, Dinner, Side Dishes, and Desserts. (I created another weekly menu as an example and inspiration for you.) Just remember that you can have three meals and two mini-meals per day, between 7:00 a.m. and 7:30 p.m., and either your lunch or dinner must be vegetarian. I also have a selection of Acid Watcher–friendly side dishes if you want to make substitutions, or if you have a dessert craving you can't shake. In either case, plan your meals for the week in advance, and use the weekly shopping list to be stocked with Acid Watcher–friendly food items at all times.

All the recipes for the Healing Phase were created according to all the Acid Watcher tenets that I've described in the book and are aimed at healing acid-damaged tissue. All require a relatively short amount of time for preparation. All menu options allow for ingredient substitution, as long as the food items come from the list of foods with a pH of 5 or higher allowed in the Healing Phase. (This will allow for infinite smoothie variations!)

The meals are designed in such a way that even someone who doesn't have a lot of experience in the kitchen will be able to prepare them. Some of them are big enough for two people to share, while others are intended for a single meal. Because so many people work outside the home during the day, I also took into consideration that they don't have time for long meal preparation at lunchtime. That is why most lunches in the diet can be eaten cold and be prepared the night before. If a work or social commitment requires you to eat out, you can use the following tips to make Acid Watcher–friendly selections in just about any eatery.

How to Be an Acid Watcher at a Restaurant

The Acid Watcher Diet is designed to be portable. That means that if you don't want to bring your lunch to work, or if you conduct your business over meals at a restaurant, don't worry—just learn to read the menu and ask the chef to make minor adjustments to the dishes you select. Here are a few easy tips to remember:

1. Whether you are at a restaurant, deli, or the prepared food court of your local grocery store, buy only chicken or seafood if you want animal protein.

2. Chicken, seafood, and vegetables should be roasted, seared, broiled, steamed, baked, or grilled.

3. Skip breaded, fried, and sauced options.

4. Keep enjoying sushi, if that's your pleasure; just stay away from soy sauce and wasabi.

THE HEALING PHASE WEEKLY SHOPPING LIST

This section contains your weekly shopping list for the Healing Phase of the Acid Watcher Diet, which should be repeated for four consecutive weeks, if you are following the weekly menu. The protein, fruit, and vegetable amounts are calculated based on the needs of one person, so if multiple members of your household are on the Acid Watcher Diet, you may want to adjust the amounts accordingly.

Please note that aside from proteins, fruits, and vegetables, almost all items purchased in the first week will carry over into the following weeks of the diet.

Fish

5 to 6 ounces salmon fillet

5 to 6 ounces skinless halibut fillet

5 to 6 ounces fresh fish fillet (tilapia, trout, flounder, branzino, or sole—buy fresh for Thursday)

Poultry

1 pound boneless, skinless chicken breast

4 to 5 ounces ground turkey (buy fresh for Wednesday)

Eggs

12 eggs

Vegetables and Herbs

1 pound spinach

1 head romaine lettuce

1/4 pound arugula

1 bunch curly kale (for salad)

4 to 5 ounces (5 to 6 leaves) kale (for juicing)

1 to 2 medium heads bok choy

2 pounds broccoli

1 bunch asparagus

3 celery stalks

2 to 3 cucumbers

1 small zucchini

1 small eggplant

1 yellow squash (non-GMO)

1 small potato

2 sweet potatoes

2 pounds carrots (not baby carrots)

1 raw beet

1 piece fresh ginger

3 to 4 ounces green beans (fresh or frozen)

3 to 4 ounces organic corn (frozen, non-GMO)

1 small package green peas (frozen)

3 ounces cremini mushrooms

1 bunch basil

1 bunch cilantro

1 bunch parsley

1 small package fresh rosemary

1 small package fresh herbs such as thyme, sage, or savory

Olives

3 ounces pitted black olives

Raw Fruit

3 to 5 bananas

2 ripe Bosc pears

2 cups mixed berries (blueberries, raspberries, blackberries, strawberries)

1 papaya (non-GMO)

2¹/₂ pounds fresh fruit: cantaloupe, watermelon, honeydew, lychee

3 Hass avocados

Dried Fruit

5 pitted halawi dates

1 small package black raisins (without preservatives and coloring)

1 small package shredded coconut

Nuts and Seeds (raw, unsalted)

1 small package pecans

2 ounces your choice of cashews, pecans, or pistachios

1 small package walnuts

1 small package pumpkin seeds (pepitas)

1 small package sesame seeds

1 small package almonds

1 small package pine nuts

Spreads

1 small container fresh, raw, organic peanut butter

1 small container fresh almond butter

Cheese

¹/₂ pound crumpled feta cheese

¹/₂ pound fresh buffalo mozzarella

4 ounces grated Parmesan cheese

Nondairy Milk

¹/₂ gallon nondairy milk, either soy milk (non-GMO) or rice milk

¹/₂ gallon almond milk (unsweetened)

Breads and Grains

1 small package either steel-cut or old-fashioned rolled oats

1 small package whole-grain fusilli pasta

1 loaf 100% whole-grain bread

1 small package whole-wheat flour

Condiments

1 package Celtic salt

1 bottle extra virgin olive oil or coconut oil

1 bottle Bragg Liquid Aminos

1 small package hemp protein (optional for smoothies)

1 small bottle vanilla extract

A COMPLETE LIST OF PH 5 FOODS ALLOWED DURING THE HEALING PHASE

If, after following the menu plan for a week or two, you decide that you want to create your own menu, the following is a list of the allowed food items:

pH 5 Raw Vegetables and Herbs

English cucumber	7.6
Zucchini	6.8
Cauliflower	6.72
Romaine lettuce	6.6
Spinach	6.5
Broccoli	6.28
Celery	6.24
Iceberg lettuce	6.23
Swiss chard (raw)	6.22
Asparagus (raw)	6.21
Cilantro (fresh)	6.18
Kale	6.01
Cabbage	5.98
Arugula	5.92
Basil	5.92
Parsley (fresh)	5.65
Garden cucumber	5.44
Orange bell pepper	5.2

pH 5 Raw and Dried Fruits

Avocado	7.12
Black olives (Cerignola, in water)	7.10
Watermelon	6.53
Cantaloupe	6.42
Lychee	5.91
Butternut squash (raw)	5.81
Banana	5.71
Papaya	5.66
Dates (halawi, Delilah)	5.49

Turkish apricot	5.1
Dragon fruit	5.45
Honeydew	5.42
Pumpkin	5.40
Bosc pear	5.15

pH 5 Root Vegetables

Cremini mushrooms	6.79
Redskin potato (cooked)	6.4
Ginger	6.28
Leeks	6.21
Beets (raw)	6.19
Carrots (raw)	6.14
Garlic	6.17
Onion (sweet)	6.15
Potato (Russet or Yukon Gold, cooked)	5.95
Sweet potato (cooked)	5.91
Carrots (cooked)	5.83
Beets (cooked)	5.79

pH 5 Dairy Products

Blue cheese	6.99
Butter (salted)	5.86
Hard cheese (Dublin)	5.8
Hard cheese (Parmesan)	5.4
Hard cheese (Asiago)	5.20
Soft cheese (mozzarella)	5.2
Hard cheese (Cheddar)	5.16

pH 5 Eggs

Egg white	8.84
Egg (hard-boiled, organic)	7.48
Egg yolk	6.32

pH 5 Dairy Alternatives

Almond milk (vanilla, Silk)	8.40
Almond milk (original flavor, Silk)	8.36
Soy milk (plain)	7.94
Tofu	6.9
Rice milk (plain, organic)	6.35

pH 5 Tree Nuts

Almonds (raw)	6.08
Walnuts (raw)	5.96
Cashews (salted)	5.41
Pistachios (salted)	5.33

pH 5 Condiments and Spreads

Almond butter (natural)	6.32
Peanut butter (fresh ground)	6.15
Bragg Liquid Aminos (soy sauce alternative)	5.00

pH 5 Waters

Evamor	8.8
Aquadeco	7.78
Jana	7.78
Smart Water	7.7
Fuji	7.55
Evian	7.36
Arizona Vapor Water	7.3

NYC tap water (unfiltered)	7.23
Voss flat water	6.68
NYC tap water (filtered—Multipure)	6.59
Perrier	5.64
Dasani	5.46
Coconut water (Zico)	5.2
Distilled water	5.22

pH 5 Meats, Poultry, Fish, and Seafood

Lobster (boiled)	7.30
Shrimp (boiled)	6.92
Crabmeat	6.75
Halibut (poached)	6.62
Salmon (grilled)	6.32
Octopus (grilled)	6.30
Tuna (in water, canned)	6.18
Turkey (fresh, roasted)	6.17
Sardines (fresh)	6.15
Tuna (seared)	6.10
Cod (broiled)	6.05
Hamburger meat	5.8
Chicken (grilled)	5.23
Beef (sirloin)	5.1

pH 5 Breads

Multigrain bread (Bread Alone)	5.53
Ezekiel 4:9 Flax	5.48
100% whole-grain bread	5.35
Ezekiel 4:9 Sesame	5.27
Whole-wheat fiber bread	5.07

pH 5 Legumes

Peas (green)	6.80
Peas (black-eyed)	6.62
Edamame	6.57
Cannellini (canned, organic)	6.10
Beans (canned, garbanzo, Goya)	6.04
Beans (canned, black, Goya)	5.93
Beans (canned, red, Goya)	5.87

THE HEALING PHASE WEEKLY MEAL PLAN

This is the weekly meal plan for the Healing Phase that I have devised for my patients. Each meal and mini-meal has a designation to help you see how it is balanced:

AP = Animal Protein dish (fish or poultry)

V = Vegetarian dish

G = Grain

F = Fruit

E/D = Eggs or Dairy

Snacks

V = Vegetarian

F = Fruit

E/D = Eggs or Dairy

N = Nut-based

N/F = Nuts and Fruit

If you choose to follow this schedule of meals, I suggest that you keep a copy of it on your refrigerator door to keep you on track. Most patients followed this menu for Week 1 for four consecutive weeks and didn't feel the need to devise their own. If, however, you like more variety week by week, feel free to plan your own meals from the Acid Watcher recipes in this section, keeping in mind that one of your daily meals—lunch or dinner—should be vegetarian.

HEALING PHASE WEEK 1 MEAL PLAN

	DAY 1	DAY 2	DAY 3	DAY 4	DAY 5	DAY 6	DAY 7
Breakfast 7–9 a.m.	F Dr. Aviv's Berry Smoothie Blast (p. 158)	E/D Spinach Omelet (p. 161)	G Banana Oatmeal (p. 161)	F Dr. Aviv's Berry Smoothie Blast (p. 158)	E/D Broccoli Omelet (p. 162)	G Pear Oatmeal (p. 162)	V Green Juice (p. 158)
Morning Mini-Meal 10–11 a.m.	V Guac Tapenade Toast (p. 164)	F Fresh fruit (8 ounces)	V Raw veggies	E/D Hard-boiled egg	F Fresh fruit (8 ounces)	E/D Mozzarella Herb Toast (p. 164)	N Toast with almond butter and honey
Lunch 12:30–2:00 p.m.	AP Dr. Aviv's Healthy Chicken Nuggets (p. 166) and asparagus	V High-Fiber Salad (p. 166)	AP Pesto Chicken Sandwich (p. 167)	V Kale Wrap with Guac Tapenade (p. 168)	V Vegetable Pasta Salad (p. 169)	AP Colorful Chicken Salad (p. 170)	AP Broiled Herbed Salmon with Steamed Spinach (p. 171)
Afternoon Mini-Meal 3–4 p.m.	N/F Dr. Aviv's Power Bar (p. 165)	N Assorted tree nuts	F Fresh fruit (6–7 ounces)	N Toast with almond butter	N Assorted tree nuts	F Fresh fruit (5–6 ounces)	F Fresh fruit (8 ounces)
Dinner 6–7:30 p.m.	V Kale "Cobb" Salad (p. 227)	AP Miso-Agave-Glazed Halibut with Sesame Bok Choy (p. 174)	V Cream of Broccoli Soup with Pepitas and Sweet Potato Fries (p. 185)	AP Turkey Burger with Arugula-Ginger Salad (p. 175)	AP Fish and Chips (p. 176)	V Papaya Salad (p. 177)	V Roasted Vegetable Sandwich (p. 178)

Following is an example of what the second week on the Healing Phase might look like. Whether you choose my plans or construct your own following the guidelines of the Healing Phase, I suggest you plan your meals in advance, which will make it easier to stick to the program.

HEALING PHASE WEEK 2 MEAL PLAN

	DAY 1	DAY 2	DAY 3	DAY 4	DAY 5	DAY 6	DAY 7
Breakfast 7–9 a.m.	N "Chocolate" Almond Butter Cup Smoothie (p. 159)	G High-Fiber Rice Pudding (p. 163)	F Dr. Aviv's Berry Smoothie Blast (p. 158)	G Pear Oatmeal (p. 162)	F Dr. Aviv's Berry Smoothie Blast (p. 158)	E/D Broccoli Omelet (p. 162)	N "Chocolate" Almond Butter Cup Smoothie (p. 159)
Morning Mini-Meal 10–11 a.m.	F Fresh fruit (8 ounces)	V Raw veggies	E/D Mozzarella Herb Toast (p. 164)	N/F Dr. Aviv's Power Bar (p. 165)	V Guac Tapenade Toast (p. 164)	F Fresh fruit (8 ounces)	E/D Mozzarella Herb Toast (p. 164)
Lunch 12:30–2:00 p.m.	G High-Fiber Salad (p. 166)	AP Colorful Chicken Salad (p. 170)	V Vegetable Pasta Salad (p. 169)	AP Mexican Shrimp Salad with Avocado, Black Beans, and Cilantro (p. 179)	AP Dr. Aviv's Healthy Chicken Nuggets (p. 166) with $1/2$ pound of ph 5 vegetables, raw or steamed	V Roasted Vegetable Sandwich (p. 178)	AP Turkey Burger with Arugula-Ginger Salad (p. 175)
Afternoon Mini-Meal 3–4 p.m.	V Raw veggies	F Fresh fruit (8 ounces)	N Assorted tree nuts	V Raw veggies	N Assorted tree nuts	N/F Dr. Aviv's Power Bar (p. 165)	V Raw veggies
Dinner 6–7:30 p.m.	AP Broiled Herbed Salmon with Steamed Spinach (p. 171)	V Kale Wrap with Guac Tapenade (p. 168)	AP Miso-Agave-Glazed Halibut with Sesame Bok Choy (p. 174)	V Roasted Beets and Fresh Cucumber with Creamy White Bean Dip (p. 182)	F Papaya Salad (p. 177)	F Fish and Chips (p. 176)	V Beet and Quinoa Salad with Steamed Kale and Chickpeas (p. 183)

Recipes for the Healing Phase

The recipes are organized in five categories for easy reference—Breakfast, Mini-Meals, Lunch, Dinner, Side Dishes (to be paired with fish or poultry meals), and Desserts, if the craving strikes you. As the Healing Phase requires you to follow the Rule of 5, you can refer to pages 150–154 for a complete list of ingredients that have a pH value of 5 and higher allowed during the Healing Phase of the diet.

HEALING PHASE BREAKFAST RECIPES

DR. AVIV'S BERRY SMOOTHIE BLAST (F)
Serves 1   Prep time: 5 minutes

This smoothie is a favorite among my patients. Remember that berries must be neutralized by nondairy nut or coconut milks to be in line with the Acid Watcher guidelines. Feel free to throw in spinach or 1 tablespoon hemp protein for an even stronger nutrient blast.

    1 cup blueberries or mixed berries
    $1/2$ cup almond milk
    1 banana
    3 to 4 ice cubes (optional)

Place the ingredients in a blender and blend until smooth. Pour into a glass and serve.

GREEN JUICE (V)
Serves 1 (12 to 15 ounces)   Prep time: 5 to 10 minutes

You need a juicer to make this recipe in your own kitchen, but if you don't have one, you can still enjoy this juice at one of your local juice bars. Just ask your server to make the juice using the green ingredients that you've selected, as they have to be nonacidic. You can add or substitute the following vegetables for the green juice: beets, bok choy, parsley, cilantro, Swiss chard, and lettuce. If you want it on the sweeter side, just add more carrots.

    2 to 3 large carrots
    5 to 6 leaves kale
    2 organic celery stalks
    1 ripe Bosc pear or $1/2$ cup any other fruit above pH 5
    1 organic cucumber

1 cup organic fresh spinach

3 to 4 ice cubes

Put all of the fruits and vegetables in a juicer and process. Pour into a glass, add a few cubes of ice, and sip slowly.

"CHOCOLATE" ALMOND BUTTER CUP SMOOTHIE (G)

Serves 2   Prep time: 5 minutes

Who can beat the simplicity of placing the ingredients in the blender, pushing a button, and producing a quick refreshing breakfast or snack?

$1/4$ cup rolled oats

$1/2$ teaspoon vanilla extract

1 tablespoon carob powder

1 tablespoon almond butter

1 banana

1 cup almond milk

2 ice cubes

Place the ingredients in a blender and blend until smooth. Pour into a glass and serve.

ACID WATCHER BLUEBERRY CREPES (G)

Serves 3   Prep and cooking time: 20 minutes

It takes a while to attain proficiency in crepe making, so don't get discouraged if your first effort goes bust. Just keep trying. Depending on the size of the crepe pan, each serving has two to four crepes.

CREPES

1 large egg

1 cup almond milk

Pinch of Celtic salt

1 teaspoon agave nectar

2 to 3 drops vanilla extract (optional)

1 cup whole-grain flour

1 tablespoon coconut oil, plus more for greasing the pan

FILLING

1 cup fresh blueberries

2 teaspoons agave nectar

In a large bowl, whisk the egg, almond milk, salt, agave nectar, vanilla (if using), and 1/2 cup water. Add the flour and whisk thoroughly, making sure there are no lumps in the batter. If the batter seems thick, dilute with more milk or water, a teaspoon at a time. Whisk in the oil.

Heat a medium nonstick pan over high heat. Using a pastry brush, grease the pan with a drizzle of oil. Use a ladle to pour the batter into the pan, moving the pan to make sure that the batter spreads evenly over the surface. Once the batter is spread out evenly, place the pan back on the stove, reduce the heat to medium, and cook the crepe until the edges become firm, 60 to 90 seconds. Flip the crepe using a thin, flat spatula, and cook for 1 minute more.

Remove the crepe to a plate. Repeat the process until all of the batter has been used, continuing to grease the pan with more oil if it gets too dry.

Make the filling: In a medium saucepan, bring the blueberries and agave nectar to a boil. Reduce to a simmer. Gently mash the berries with a spatula to help them release their juices. Simmer for 5 to 10 minutes, until the fruit reduces to a desired thickness, and remove from the heat.

To serve, lay a crepe on a plate and add a tablespoon of the filling to the middle. Wrap it up either into a triangle or a roll. Repeat the process with the remaining crepes and filling. Serve immediately.

SPINACH OMELET (AP)

Serves 1   Prep time: 5 to 10 minutes

This diner favorite is easy to make for breakfast, lunch, or dinner, if you are hungry but not enough to spend more than 5 or 10 minutes in the kitchen.

> $1/2$ teaspoon olive or coconut oil
>
> 1 large egg
>
> 2 large egg whites
>
> 1 tablespoon chopped black olives
>
> 1 teaspoon grated Parmesan cheese (optional)
>
> Handful of fresh spinach
>
> 1 slice toasted whole-grain bread

Heat the oil in a pan over medium-low heat. In a small bowl, whisk the egg and the egg whites with the olives and Parmesan (if using). Pour the egg mixture into the pan, and when it starts to sizzle but before it is cooked all the way through, add the spinach and stir for 1 minute more, or until the eggs are cooked through. Remove from the heat and serve with the whole-grain toast.

BANANA OATMEAL WITH PECANS
AND COCONUT FLAKES (G)

Serves 1   Prep and cooking time: 5 to 10 minutes

You'll never miss the high-sugar, acid-loaded breakfast cereals if you master this filling comfort breakfast.

> $1/2$ cup nondairy milk (organic soy milk, almond milk, or rice milk)
>
> Pinch of Celtic salt
>
> 5 tablespoons old-fashioned rolled oats
>
> $1/2$ banana, sliced
>
> 1 tablespoon chopped raw pecans
>
> 1 tablespoon coconut flakes
>
> 2 to 3 drops vanilla extract (optional)

Heat the nondairy milk and salt in a nonstick pan over medium heat. Add the oats and cook, stirring constantly, until thick and creamy, about 2 minutes. Remove from the heat and add the banana, pecans, coconut flakes, and vanilla (if using). Mix well and serve.

BROCCOLI OMELET (E/D)

Serves 1   Prep and cooking time: 5 to 10 minutes

Any sturdy green vegetable can be paired with eggs, but this one is a quick and reliable classic.

- 1 large egg
- 2 large egg whites
- $1/2$ teaspoon olive or coconut oil
- Handful of chopped broccoli, room temperature
- 1 teaspoon grated Parmesan cheese
- 1 slice toasted whole-grain bread

In a small bowl, whisk the egg and egg whites. In a nonstick pan, heat the oil over medium heat. Add the broccoli to the pan and sauté for about 1 minute. Add the egg mixture and Parmesan and cook, stirring slightly, until the eggs are fluffy, about 1 minute more. When the eggs are cooked to your liking, remove from the heat and serve with the whole-grain toast.

PEAR OATMEAL WITH PECANS
AND COCONUT FLAKES (G)

Serves 1   Prep and cooking time: 5 to 10 minutes

- $1/2$ cup nondairy milk (organic soy milk, almond milk, or rice milk)
- Pinch of Celtic salt
- 5 tablespoons old-fashioned rolled oats
- 2 to 3 drops vanilla extract (optional)
- $1/2$ Bosc pear, ripe, cut into small chunks

1 tablespoon chopped raw pecans or walnuts

1 tablespoon coconut flakes

In a small saucepan, heat the nondairy milk and salt over medium heat. Add the oats and vanilla (if using) and cook, stirring constantly, until thick and creamy, 2 to 3 minutes. Remove from the heat, stir in the pear chunks, pecans, and coconut flakes, and serve.

HIGH-FIBER RICE PUDDING (G)
Serves 2
Prep time: 10 to 12 minutes, plus more for cooking the rice

We are accustomed to thinking of rice pudding as a dessert, but it is a perfectly viable breakfast option. And rice with dried fruit is an ideal combination for those who crave something sweet with their breakfast.

$1/2$ cup cooked brown rice

$1/2$ cup soy milk

1 teaspoon vanilla extract (optional)

$1^1/2$ tablespoons shredded coconut

2 tablespoons raisins

3 to 4 dried Turkish apricots, chopped

In a nonstick pot, combine the rice and soy milk and bring to a boil, stirring constantly. Add the vanilla (if using) and cook for 2 to 3 minutes more. Remove from the heat and stir in the coconut, raisins, and apricots. Serve immediately.

HEALING PHASE MINI-MEALS

GUAC TAPENADE TOAST (V)
Serves 1   Prep time: 5 minutes

12 pitted black olives, drained

1 ripe Hass avocado, pitted and scooped

1 teaspoon finely chopped fresh cilantro

1 slice toasted whole-grain bread

$1/3$ cucumber, peeled, seeded (if desired), and finely chopped

Handful of arugula

In a food processor, combine the olives, avocado, and cilantro and pulse until smooth. Spread the tapenade on the whole-grain toast, top with the cucumber and arugula, and serve.

MOZZARELLA HERB TOAST (D)
Serves 1   Prep time: 5 minutes

A recipe for a mini-meal doesn't get much simpler than for an open sandwich like this one.

1 slice toasted whole-grain bread

1 to 2 thin slices fresh mozzarella (approximately 1 inch in
   diameter)

2 fresh basil leaves

Top the whole-grain toast with the mozzarella slices and basil and serve.

DR. AVIV'S POWER BAR (N)

Serves 1   Prep time: 15 minutes, plus more for cooling

$2^1/2$ pitted dates

10 almonds

$1^1/2$ teaspoons organic raw peanut butter

1 drop vanilla extract

$1^1/2$ teaspoons shredded coconut

Place the dates and almonds in a food processor and pulse for about 1 minute, until the mixture is reduced to a paste. Transfer the mixture to a small mixing bowl and combine with the peanut butter and vanilla. Mix well with a spoon for 1 minute. Turn the mixture out onto a cutting board and shape it to resemble a standard "power" bar. Coat the bar with shredded coconut on both sides and enjoy one of the healthiest power bars you'll ever eat!

Note: These bars will taste even better after you cool them in the refrigerator.

FRESH FRUIT (8 OUNCES)

Choose from cantaloupe, papaya, watermelon, honeydew, ripe pear, banana, or lychee. Prepare approximately 2 cups of fruit of your choice, or a blend of any of those listed here.

ASSORTED TREE NUTS

An ounce of tree nuts is about a handful. Choose your favorites from walnuts, cashews, pecans, or pistachios.

RAW VEGGIES

Slice a carrot, a celery stick, and half of an English cucumber. You can use a pinch of Celtic salt to flavor, if necessary.

HEALING PHASE LUNCH RECIPES

DR. AVIV'S HEALTHY CHICKEN NUGGETS (A/P)
Serves 1   Prep and cooking time: 15 to 20 minutes

    1 large egg
    Celtic salt, to taste
    2 tablespoons whole-wheat flour
    4 to 5 ounces boneless, skinless chicken breast
    $1/2$ teaspoon chopped fresh rosemary
    1 teaspoon chopped fresh parsley
    $1/2$ teaspoon olive or coconut oil

Prepare an assembly line. In a small bowl, whisk the egg with a pinch of salt. Place a bowl with the flour next to it. Slice the chicken breast into four equal pieces. Season with salt, rosemary, and parsley. Cover the chicken pieces with plastic wrap and pound on each side to tenderize.

In a nonstick pan, heat the oil over medium heat. Moving quickly, dip the chicken into the egg, one piece at a time, then transfer it to the bowl with flour, coating the piece on both sides. Carefully place the chicken piece into the pan. Repeat with the other three pieces. Cook the chicken for 2 to 3 minutes on each side. Add 2 tablespoons of water, cover the pan, and cook for 2 to 3 minutes more, until all the water evaporates. If you like your chicken crispy, cook for an extra minute or two.

HIGH-FIBER SALAD (V)
Serves 1   Prep time: 5 to 10 minutes

This is a go-to Acid Watcher fresh vegetable salad. See instructions on how to blanch peas on page 135, and how to roast beets on page 182, if you would prefer to consume these ingredients cooked. Feel free to use any other vegetable measuring pH 5 or higher in this recipe. In the Maintenance Phase, you can add bell peppers to the mix.

2 to 3 ounces (3 large leaves) romaine lettuce, chopped

Handful of chopped raw broccoli

1/2 cup chopped cucumber

3 tablespoons shredded carrot

5 to 6 pitted kalamata olives, drained and chopped

3 tablespoons fresh or frozen green peas, blanched

3 tablespoons shredded raw or roasted beets

1 teaspoon olive oil

2 tablespoons crumbled feta cheese

Pinch of Celtic salt (optional)

1 slice whole-grain bread, toasted and cubed (optional)

Place all the ingredients in a salad bowl and mix.

PESTO CHICKEN SANDWICH (AP)
Serves 1   Prep and cooking time: 20 minutes

This rustic, tasty chicken sandwich is so easy to make that you'll forget about ever going back to your local deli. If you don't have the time to roast your own piece of chicken, buy one from a trusted rotisserie. Just make sure to get a plain, roasted chicken, not one that was marinated in lemon, garlic, teriyaki, or any other processed mix.

4 to 5 ounces boneless, skinless chicken breast, or leftover chicken from Homemade Chicken Broth (page 229), if available

Pinch of Celtic salt

1/4 cup plus 1 tablespoon organic olive oil

2 cups fresh basil leaves, tightly packed

1/4 cup unsalted pine nuts

2 tablespoons grated Parmesan cheese (optional)

2 slices whole-grain bread

2 leaves romaine lettuce or a handful of arugula

2 thin slices fresh buffalo mozzarella

To prepare the boneless, skinless chicken breast, preheat the oven to 400°F. Sprinkle the chicken with salt and coat it in 1 tablespoon of the oil. Roast in a roasting pan or on a baking sheet lined with parchment paper for 12 to 15 minutes, turning the chicken over once about halfway through the process. Remove from the oven and allow to cool completely.

While the chicken is roasting, make the pesto by pulsing the basil leaves, the remaining 1/4 cup oil, pine nuts, and Parmesan (if using) in a food processor until the mixture reaches a claylike consistency.

Chop the chicken into bite-size pieces. Combine with a tablespoon of the pesto in a bowl, stirring gently to make sure all the pieces are coated. Line the bread slices with the lettuce and mozzarella. Spoon the pesto chicken on top and enjoy, as either an open or a closed sandwich.

The leftover pesto can be frozen for up to 1 month.

Modifications and additions: For a nondairy version of the sauce, omit the Parmesan and mozzarella. Add more salt if needed.

KALE WRAP WITH GUAC TAPENADE (V)
Serves 1   Prep time: 10 to 12 minutes

This dish is a pure explosion of nutrients in a wrap. Just remember that it has to be consumed immediately, as the avocado oxidizes quickly without citrus.

    12 pitted black olives, drained
    1 ripe Hass avocado, pitted and scooped
    1 teaspoon fresh cilantro leaves
    2 to 3 leaves fresh kale, washed, dried, stems removed
    1/3 cucumber, peeled, seeded, and finely chopped
    Handful of arugula

In a food processor, pulse the olives, avocado, and cilantro to make the tapenade. Spread the tapenade on the kale leaves and top with cucumber and arugula. Roll up the kale leaves and enjoy right away!

VEGETABLE PASTA SALAD (V)

Serves 1   Prep and cooking time: 20 minutes

You'll never go back to the popular restaurant-style pasta primavera if you master this easy dish. It is even delicious cold!

Celtic salt, to taste
1/2 cup whole-grain fusilli pasta
5 to 6 asparagus stalks
3 ounces cremini mushrooms
1 teaspoon olive oil
1 tablespoon chopped fresh parsley
1 handful fresh arugula, roughly chopped
2 teaspoons grated Parmesan cheese

Bring a large pot of salted water to a rapid boil over high heat. Add the pasta and cook for approximately 9 minutes, until al dente. Remove from the heat and drain.

While the pasta is cooking, prepare the asparagus, washing each stalk thoroughly and trimming the ends (see Note). Cut the asparagus into 1/2-inch segments. Wash and dry the mushrooms and slice them into chunks.

In a heavy-bottomed pan, heat the oil over high heat. Add the mushrooms, reduce the heat to medium, and sauté for about 3 minutes, or until the mushrooms begin to brown around the edges. Sprinkle with salt. Add the asparagus and parsley. Sauté for about 3 minutes, stirring occasionally.

Remove the vegetables from the pan and mix into the pasta. Add the arugula and Parmesan, mix well, and enjoy a wonderful vegetarian pasta meal.

Note: The expert way to trim asparagus is to hold a stalk in your hands on both ends, bend it inward, and allow it to snap. It is going to break naturally at a spot where the tender flesh ends and the fibrous part begins. Some cooks yelp when they see how much of the asparagus is lost in this process, but it will be more satisfying in texture without the woody part. The asparagus ends need not be wasted though, as they are full of nutrients. Freeze them and use them when preparing homemade stocks and soups.

COLORFUL CHICKEN SALAD (AP)

Serves 1   Prep and cooking time: 25 minutes

For this recipe you can use frozen vegetables, and if you didn't defrost them in advance, you can blanch them for 2 to 3 minutes. This chicken salad can be versatile, as it goes with just about any vegetable. Once you have graduated to the Maintenance Phase of the diet, you can make it more colorful by adding $1/2$ roasted red bell pepper, chopped, and 2 tablespoons finely chopped raw leeks.

> Celtic salt, to taste
> 1 teaspoon olive oil
> 4 to 5 ounces boneless, skinless chicken breast
> 3 to 4 ounces frozen organic corn, thawed
> 3 to 4 ounces frozen green beans, thawed and finely chopped
> 2 to 3 tablespoons Bragg Liquid Aminos
> 1 tablespoon honey
> Dash of Celtic salt (optional)

Preheat the oven to 400°F. Sprinkle the salt and oil over the chicken and roast in a pan or on a baking sheet lined with parchment paper for 10 to 12 minutes, flipping the chicken over once halfway through the cooking process. Remove from the oven, allow to cool completely, and chop into small cubes.

In a medium bowl, mix the chicken with the corn and beans and coat with Bragg Liquid Aminos, honey, and salt to taste (if using).

BROILED HERBED SALMON WITH
STEAMED SPINACH (AP)

Serves 1   Prep and cooking time: 12 to 15 minutes

You can use fresh or frozen salmon fillet for this recipe. If you are using frozen salmon, make sure it is fully defrosted and dried with a paper towel before you cook it.

> 1 tablespoon plus 1 teaspoon olive oil
>
> 5 ounces salmon fillet, skin on
>
> 2 pinches of Celtic salt
>
> 1 teaspoon herbs (fresh or dried parsley, thyme, sage, or rosemary)
>
> 2 to 3 lemon slices
>
> 2 cups fresh baby spinach

In a thick-bottomed pan, heat 1 tablespoon of the oil over medium-low heat for about 1 minute. Pour $1/4$ cup water into the pan and bring to a simmer. Place the salmon in the pan, skin side up, and add a pinch of salt and $1/2$ teaspoon of the herbs. Cover the pan and cook for 2 to 3 minutes. Turn the fillet over and top with the lemon slices. Add more water if needed. Sprinkle with the remaining $1/2$ teaspoon herbs and cook, covered, for another 2 to 3 minutes. If you want your salmon crispy and well done, allow it to cook for 1 to 2 minutes more after the water evaporates. Keep an eye on the salmon to prevent burning.

While the salmon is cooking, heat the remaining 1 teaspoon oil in a separate pan. Add the spinach and a pinch of salt and sauté for about 2 minutes, until the spinach wilts and the water that it releases evaporates.

Plate the salmon fillet on top of the spinach and serve.

Modifications and additions: If you'd like, enjoy with $1/2$ slice toasted whole-grain bread.

SALMON SPINACH SALAD WITH SLICED PEARS, WALNUTS, AND OLIVES (AP)

Serves 2

Prep and cooking time: 15 to 20 minutes,
more if using dried beans

You can use either dried or canned chickpeas for this recipe. If you cook your own chickpeas, feel free to make more than the recipe calls for. You can store the leftovers in your refrigerator for up to a week and mix with other salads. Be careful not to scorch the salmon fillets in the broiler; they'll cook faster on the surface if you place them closer to the flame, but the inside may be undercooked. Keep the salmon away from direct flame if you want the fillets broiled more evenly throughout.

$1/2$ cup dried chickpeas, or 1 cup canned chickpeas

2 (4-ounce) salmon fillets, skin on

1 teaspoon olive oil, plus more for drizzling

Celtic salt, to taste

4 cups fresh baby spinach

1 ripe medium Bosc pear, thinly sliced into $1/2$-inch pieces

$1/2$ cup walnuts, toasted and roughly chopped

$1/2$ cup golden raisins

$1/4$ cup pitted kalamata olives, drained and chopped

$1/4$ cup pitted green olives, drained

For freshly cooked chickpeas, rinse the $1/2$ cup dried chickpeas, cover with water in a large glass bowl, and soak overnight. Rinse thoroughly. Bring to a boil in 2 cups salted water, then reduce the heat to medium. Cover and simmer for 40 to 45 minutes, until the chickpeas are tender and before they start falling apart. Drain and cool to room temperature. (If you use canned beans, please make sure the product is organic. Organic canned beans should contain only water, salt, and beans. To use canned beans for this recipe, simply open the can, rinse the beans well, and add them to the recipe.)

Preheat the broiler. Place the salmon on an aluminum or parchment-lined baking sheet, drizzle with oil, sprinkle with salt, and broil until golden brown, about 5 to 7 minutes. Remove from the oven and allow to cool completely.

Toss the chickpeas, spinach, pear, walnuts, raisins, and olives with 1 teaspoon oil and salt. Plate the salads on two plates, top each with a salmon fillet, and serve.

HEALING PHASE DINNER RECIPES

MISO-AGAVE-GLAZED HALIBUT
WITH SESAME BOK CHOY (AP)
Serves 1   Prep and cooking time: 15 to 20 minutes

This dish is very light, delicate, and exotic. If you don't have access to halibut (it is a seasonal dish), cod or any thick-fleshed white fish would be a good substitute.

> 1 tablespoon white miso
> $1/2$ teaspoon agave nectar
> 5 to 6 ounces halibut fillet, boneless and skinless
> $1/2$ teaspoon organic olive oil, plus more for the pan
> 1 to 2 medium heads bok choy, roughly chopped
> Pinch of Celtic salt
> $1/2$ teaspoon sesame seeds
> $1/2$ slice toasted whole-grain bread (optional)

Preheat the broiler. In a medium bowl, whisk the miso, agave nectar, and 1 to 2 tablespoons water. Place the halibut in the mixture and marinate for 15 minutes. Place on a pan lined with oiled foil and broil for 5 to 7 minutes, until the edges of the fillet are caramelized to golden brown.

While the fish is broiling, in a large sauté pan, heat $1/2$ teaspoon oil over medium heat. Add the bok choy and salt. Sauté for 1 to 2 minutes, until tender. Sprinkle with sesame seeds.

Serve with $1/2$ slice whole-grain toast (if using).

TURKEY BURGERS WITH
ARUGULA-GINGER SALAD (AP)

Serves 2   Prep and cooking time: 15 to 20 minutes

Think of these as "breadless" burgers as they are not served in a bun. But who needs a bun if all the goodness of the inside—a deliciously cooked patty and fresh vegetables—is still on the plate?

TURKEY BURGERS

$4^1/2$ ounces ground turkey (white meat, dark meat, or a
 combination)

$^1/2$ medium carrot, shredded

$^1/3$ medium celery stalk, chopped

3 tablespoons shredded zucchini, squeezed to drain excess
 liquid (optional)

1 small red potato, shredded

$^1/4$ teaspoon Celtic salt

1 small egg

2 tablespoons whole-wheat flour

1 teaspoon olive oil

Bragg Liquid Aminos

CARROT-GINGER DRESSING

$^1/2$ raw carrot, shredded

1 tablespoon organic olive oil

1 tablespoon agave nectar

$^1/4$ inch fresh ginger, peeled and coarsely chopped

$^1/4$ teaspoon Celtic salt

SALAD

$^1/2$ cup finely chopped arugula

$1^1/2$ cups fresh spinach

Make the turkey burgers: In a large bowl, combine the turkey, carrot, celery, zucchini (if using), and potato and sprinkle with salt. In a separate bowl, whisk the egg and pour half of it over the turkey mixture. (Be careful not to use all of the egg, as the turkey might become too wet.) Mix the turkey mixture thoroughly and then make 3 to 4 burgers from it. On another plate, pour out the flour and then coat each burger completely.

In a nonstick pan, heat the oil over low heat, then place the burgers in the pan. Cover and cook for 4 to 5 minutes, turning over at least once. After the burgers are cooked, remove from the heat and drizzle each burger with 1 to 2 sprays of Bragg Liquid Aminos.

Make the dressing: In a food processor, pulse the ingredients with ¼ cup water until smooth.

Make the salad: Toss the greens with the carrot-ginger dressing and serve alongside the turkey burgers.

FISH AND CHIPS (AP)

Serves 1   Prep and cooking time: 20 to 25 minutes

The classic comfort food has been revised for the Acid Watcher, with the nutritious sweet potato replacing the starchier white potato, and the preparation technique changed from deep-frying to baking. The color and the taste are still there, but the bad calories aren't.

    5 to 6 ounces fish fillet (tilapia, trout, flounder, branzino, or sole)
    Celtic salt, to taste
    2 teaspoons chopped fresh rosemary
    2 to 3 teaspoons olive oil
    2 thin lemon slices
    1 large sweet potato, peeled, washed, and cut into strips

Preheat the oven to 400°F. Sprinkle the fillet with salt and rosemary and drizzle with half of the oil. Place on a nonstick baking sheet lined with a generous sheet of foil. Place the lemon slices on the fish and close the foil around it, creating a tight pocket.

Sprinkle the sweet potatoes with salt and drizzle with the remaining oil. Place the fries on the baking sheet with the fish on a piece of parchment paper to avoid sticking.

Bake for 15 to 20 minutes, turning the fries with a spatula every 5 minutes. When the fries become soft on the inside and a bit crunchy on the outside, remove the pan from the oven. The fish should be tender and separate into pieces easily. Serve immediately.

PAPAYA SALAD (V)

Serves 1   Prep and cooking time: 12 to 15 minutes

Tangy and naturally sweet, this refreshing summer salad makes a perfect supper or a weekend lunch.

- 1 tablespoon plus 1 teaspoon organic olive oil
- 1 medium carrot, shredded
- 1 tablespoon agave nectar
- $1/4$ inch fresh ginger, peeled and coarsely chopped
- $1/4$ teaspoon Celtic salt
- 1 large kale leaf (about 12 inches), stem removed, chopped
- 3 teaspoons finely chopped walnuts
- $1/3$ English cucumber, chopped
- 10 to 15 raisins, chopped
- 2 tablespoons crumbled feta cheese
- $1/2$ cup papaya (non-GMO), peeled and cut into $1/2$-inch cubes

To make the salad dressing, in a food processor, pulse the oil and half of the carrot with the agave nectar, ginger, salt, and $1/4$ cup water for about 1 minute, until the mixture reaches a smooth consistency.

In a large bowl, combine the remaining carrot with the kale, walnuts, cucumber, and raisins. Drizzle with the dressing, mix well, and top with feta cheese and papaya cubes. Serve immediately.

ROASTED VEGETABLE SANDWICH (V)
Serves 2   Prep and cooking time: 20 minutes

This light gourmet sandwich is a great way to load up on your veggies. Because you are using only several slices of each vegetable, expect to have some leftovers; just wrap and refrigerate the remaining pieces, reserving them for future use.

1 to 2 teaspoons organic olive oil, plus more for drizzling

$1/2$ medium yellow squash, peeled and sliced into 4 circles

$1/2$ sweet potato, peeled and sliced into 8 thin circles

2 slices eggplant, approximately $1/2$ inch thick

Celtic salt, to taste

4 slices whole-grain bread

2 slices salted mozzarella cheese

4 fresh basil leaves

Preheat the oven to 450°F. In a nonstick heavy-bottomed pan, heat the oil over medium-high heat. When the oil begins to sizzle, place the squash slices in the pan and sear for about 1 minute, until the edges begin to brown. Turn over to sear the other side for 1 to 2 minutes more.

Place the potato and eggplant slices on a baking sheet lined with parchment paper, sprinkle with salt, and drizzle with oil. Roast for 12 to 15 minutes, flipping the slices every couple of minutes. When the potato is soft enough to be pierced with a fork, remove from the oven and allow to cool.

While the vegetables are cooling, lightly toast the bread and line two of the slices with mozzarella, basil, squash, potato, and eggplant. Cover with the other slices of bread and enjoy.

Note: When you get to the Maintenance Phase of the Acid Watcher Diet, you may add roasted red bell pepper.

MEXICAN SHRIMP SALAD WITH AVOCADO, BLACK BEANS, AND CILANTRO (AP)
Serves 2 to 4
Prep and cooking time: 20 to 25 minutes, more if using dried beans

This salad is a potluck crowd pleaser, but it doesn't have to be reserved for special occasions. A breeze to cook and to assemble, it will tickle your palate and fill your stomach. As everyone south of the border knows, shrimp with avocado is a match made in heaven. Shrimp is a good source of protein, and avocado is a healthy fat. The shrimp, like almost all shellfish, is the acid neutralizer in this dish, and pepitas (pumpkin seeds), the wonder seeds of Mexican cuisine, make it especially jazzy. Make extra shrimp and reserve it for batch two the next day. Believe me, you'll want it.

$3/4$ cup dried black beans, or $1^1/2$ cups canned beans

$1/2$ teaspoon Celtic salt, plus a pinch for the beans

1 jumbo romaine heart, chopped

$1/2$ English cucumber, sliced

1 ripe Hass avocado, pitted, scooped, and sliced

2 tablespoons raw pepitas

$1/2$ cup fresh cilantro, roughly chopped

3 teaspoons olive oil

$1/2$ pound jumbo shrimp, cleaned and deveined

Rinse the dried black beans, if using, and clean thoroughly. Place the beans in a large bowl, cover with water, and let soak overnight.

The next day, drain and rinse the beans, then put them in a medium saucepan and cover them with water. Add a big pinch of salt, bring to a boil, cover, and reduce to a simmer. Cook for 40 to 50 minutes, or until soft but not mushy. Drain and rinse well. Let cool. (Canned beans may be used as long as the product is organic. Organic canned beans should contain only water, salt, and beans. To use canned beans for this recipe, simply open the can, rinse the beans well, and add them to your meal.)

In a large bowl, toss the romaine, cucumber, black beans, avocado, pepitas, cilantro, 2 teaspoons of the oil, and $1/4$ teaspoon of the Celtic salt.

Heat a large sauté pan over medium heat. In a medium bowl, toss the shrimp with $1/2$ teaspoon of the oil and the remaining $1/4$ teaspoon salt. Place the shrimp in the pan in an even layer and add the remaining $1/2$ teaspoon oil and sear for 1 to 2 minutes per side, until fully cooked. Remove from the heat.

Divide the salad among your serving plates, top with the shrimp, and serve.

ACID WATCHER NIÇOISE SALAD (AP)

Serves 2   Prep and cooking time: 12 to 15 minutes

Don't ruin a perfectly delicious (and expensive) tuna steak by serving it well done. You'll destroy the flavor and the texture. Sushi-quality tuna is safe to eat rare.

$2^1/2$ teaspoons olive oil

2 (4-ounce) tuna steaks

$1/4$ teaspoon Celtic salt, plus more to taste

1 jumbo romaine lettuce leaf, chopped

2 large hard-boiled eggs, peeled and chopped

$4^1/2$ ounces green beans, trimmed, blanched, and chopped into $1/2$-inch pieces

$1/2$ cup pitted black olives, drained

1 large carrot, shredded

$1/2$ English cucumber, cut into half moons

$1/3$ cup fresh basil leaves, roughly chopped

$1/4$ cup chopped fresh parsley

Brush a nonstick sauté pan with $1/2$ teaspoon of the oil and heat over medium heat. Sprinkle both sides of each tuna steak with salt and place in the hot pan. Sear for about 1 minute on each side, until the fish is browned on the outside but rare on the inside.

Remove from the heat, bring to room temperature, and slice into strips.

Toss the romaine, eggs, green beans, olives, carrot, cucumber, basil, and parsley with the remaining 2 teaspoons oil. Divide the salad between 2 plates, sprinkle with salt, top with the seared tuna, and serve.

Modifications and additions: For a vegetarian option, omit the tuna.

HERB CHICKEN (AP)

Serves 2   Prep time: 20 minutes

The beauty of this dish is that it goes with just about any combination of vegetables, served raw, steamed, or blanched.

- 4 ounces boneless, skinless chicken breast
- 2 teaspoons olive oil
- Celtic salt, to taste
- 2 tablespoons fresh herbs (rosemary, oregano, parsley, thyme, or sage)
- 2 tablespoons whole-grain bread crumbs for sprinkling

Preheat the oven to 400°F. Slice the chicken into thin fillets, drizzle with the oil, and sprinkle with the salt and herbs. Coat in bread crumbs and place on a baking sheet lined with parchment paper.

Roast the chicken for about 15 minutes, flipping the pieces over halfway through the process. Serve with $1/2$ pound of pH 5 vegetables of your choice.

ROASTED BEETS AND FRESH CUCUMBER WITH CREAMY WHITE BEAN DIP (V)

Serves 2 to 4

Prep and cooking time: 50 minutes,

more if using dried beans

Beets are loaded with nutrients, and their natural sweetness makes for a delicious accent as a side dish, or, as in this case, a refreshing salad base. You'll get an acid neutralizer in the cucumber, a boost of fiber from the cannellini beans, and a refreshing taste from the dill.

> 1 cup dried cannellini beans, or 2 cups canned beans
>
> $3/4$ teaspoon Celtic salt, plus more to taste
>
> 1 bunch small red beets (approximately 4 small beets)
>
> $2^1/2$ teaspoons olive oil
>
> 1 tablespoon finely chopped fresh dill
>
> 1 cucumber, sliced

Rinse the dried cannellini beans and clean them thoroughly. Place the beans in a large bowl and cover with water. Let soak overnight. The next day, drain and rinse the beans, then place them in a medium saucepan and cover with water. Add a big pinch of salt, bring to a boil, cover, and reduce to a simmer. Cook for 40 to 50 minutes, or until soft but not mushy. Drain and rinse well. Let cool. (If you want to use beans from a can, please make sure the product is organic. Organic canned beans should contain only water, salt, and beans. To use canned beans for this recipe, just open the can, rinse the beans well, and add to the recipe.)

Preheat the oven to 400°F. Wash, trim, and dry the beets. Cut them in half crosswise for quicker cooking and place on a baking sheet lined with a large sheet of foil. Add 2 teaspoons of the oil and $1/4$ teaspoon of the salt. Rub in the oil and salt and evenly coat. Wrap the foil tightly around the beets. Roast until fork tender, 20 to 30 minutes, depending on the size of the beets. Let them cool, then rub with a paper towel to remove the skins. Cut into rounds.

In a food processor, combine the cannellini beans, $1/4$ cup water, the remaining $1/2$ teaspoon oil, and the remaining $1/2$ teaspoon salt. Purée until smooth, then stir in the dill.

Serve with the sliced beets and cucumbers.

BEET AND QUINOA SALAD WITH STEAMED KALE AND CHICKPEAS (V)
Serves 2 to 4
Prep time: 30 minutes, more if using dried chickpeas

For this recipe, the quinoa and chickpeas can be prepared in advance. As with all recipes that call for chickpeas, I recommend going with the dried variety, but in a pinch you can always use canned chickpeas.

- 1 cup dried chickpeas, or 2 cups canned chickpeas
- $1/4$ teaspoon Celtic salt, plus more to taste
- 1 small bunch of beets (approximately 4 small beets)
- $3^1/2$ teaspoons olive oil
- $1/2$ bunch kale (approximately 10 leaves), washed, dried, stems removed, and thinly sliced
- 1 cup cooked quinoa
- $1/4$ cup pine nuts

Rinse the dried chickpeas, picking out any stones. Place the chickpeas in a large bowl and cover completely with water. Soak the beans overnight. Drain and rinse the chickpeas, place them in a medium saucepan, and cover with water. Add a big pinch of salt, bring to a boil, cover, and reduce to a simmer. Cook for about 45 minutes, or until soft but not mushy. Drain and rinse well. Bring to room temperature. (If you want to use beans from a can, please make sure the product is organic. Organic canned beans should contain only water, salt, and beans. To use canned beans for this recipe, simply open the can, rinse the beans well, and add them to the recipe.)

While the chickpeas are cooking, make the beets: Preheat the oven to 400°F. Wash, trim, and dry the beets. Cut them in half crosswise and place them on a baking sheet lined with a large sheet of foil. Brush with 2 teaspoons of the oil and sprinkle with ¼ teaspoon of the salt. Wrap the foil tightly around the beets. Roast until fork tender, 20 to 30 minutes, depending on the size of the beets. Let cool, then rub with a paper towel to remove the skins. Chop into ¼-inch pieces.

In a medium saucepan, heat ¼ cup water. Keep the heat low and add the kale and a dash of salt. Cover and steam for 3 to 5 minutes, until the kale softens but still retains some crunch. Drain the excess water and let cool.

To serve, combine the chickpeas, beets, kale, quinoa, pine nuts, the remaining 1½ teaspoons oil, and salt to taste. Serve immediately.

PURÉED BUTTERNUT SQUASH SOUP WITH SEARED MUSHROOMS AND HERBS (V)

Serves 3   Prep and cooking time: 35 minutes

This soup is perfect comfort food on a cold day.

> 2 tablespoons olive oil
> 1 butternut squash, peeled, seeded, and cut into 1-inch cubes
> 1 teaspoon dried thyme
> 3½ to 4½ teaspoons Celtic salt
> ½ cup nondairy milk (organic soy milk, almond milk, or rice milk)
> 8 ounces cremini mushrooms, stemmed and sliced
> 2 to 3 tablespoons chopped fresh parsley

In a large pot, heat 1 tablespoon of the oil over medium heat. Add the squash, thyme, and 1½ teaspoons of the salt, and sauté for about 10 minutes, until browned and fragrant. Add 2½ cups water and bring to a boil. Cover and simmer for 10 to 12 minutes, until tender. Stir in the nondairy milk.

Transfer the squash with its liquid to a blender and purée for about 2 minutes, until smooth.

In a large sauté pan, heat the remaining 1 tablespoon oil over high heat. Once the oil is simmering, add the mushrooms in an even layer.

Cook without stirring for about 4 minutes, until golden brown. Stir and cook for another 3 to 5 minutes. Sprinkle with the remaining 2 to 3 teaspoons salt. Transfer to a plate lined with a paper towel to soak up excess oil and liquid.

To serve, divide the soup among 3 bowls and top with the seared mushrooms. Sprinkle with chopped parsley.

CREAM OF BROCCOLI SOUP WITH PEPITAS AND SWEET POTATO FRIES (DAIRY FREE) (V)
Serves 2   Prep and cooking time: 35 to 45 minutes

You can eat the soup without the sweet potato fries, but they make the meal complete and memorable.

  3 teaspoons olive oil

  3 heads broccoli, separated into florets

  2 teaspoons Celtic salt, plus more to taste

  2 cups nondairy milk (organic soy milk, almond milk, or rice milk)

  $1/2$ Hass avocado, pitted and scooped

  1 large sweet potato, peeled, washed, and cut into strips

  1 tablespoon chopped fresh rosemary

  2 tablespoons raw pepitas

In a large nonstick pot, heat 1 teaspoon of the oil over medium heat. Add the broccoli and 2 teaspoons salt. Sauté the broccoli for about 5 minutes, until it begins to soften. Add the nondairy milk and bring to a boil. Reduce to a simmer and cook for another 5 minutes.

Allow to cool slightly and transfer half of the broccoli mixture to a blender. Add the avocado and blend until smooth. Transfer the mixture into a large bowl, and the rest of the broccoli mixture into the blender. Pulse a few times to blend. This second batch of soup should retain some of its chunkiness. Combine both broccoli mixtures in the bowl.

To make the sweet potato fries, preheat the oven to 400°F. Sprinkle the fries with salt and rosemary and drizzle with 1 teaspoon of the oil. Place the fries in a single layer on a nonstick baking sheet lined with parchment paper. Bake for 15 to 20 minutes, until they become soft inside and slightly crunchy on the outside, flipping them over with a spatula or tongs every 5 minutes.

Serve the soup warm, topped with pepitas and the remaining 1 teaspoon oil, with the sweet potato fries on the side.

BROILED HERB SALMON WITH STEAMED SPINACH (AP)
Serves 1   Prep time: 12 to 15 minutes

You can enjoy this dish for a quick weekday meal. It is delicious served warm, but if you'd rather have it for lunch, it is just as satisfying served cold or at room temperature for lunch the next day.

> 5 ounces salmon fillet, skin on
> $1/2$ teaspoon Celtic salt
> $1^1/2$ teaspoons olive oil
> 1 teaspoon dried herbs (a mix of parsley, thyme, sage, rosemary)
> $1/2$ fresh lemon, sliced
> 1 cup baby spinach

Salt the salmon fillet. Heat 1 teaspoon of the olive oil in a nonstick pan on medium-high heat. Add $1/2$ cup water and bring to simmer. Place the salmon, skin side up, into the pan, add half of the herbs and lemon slices. Cover the pan and simmer for 2 to 3 minutes.

Turn the salmon over, add a splash of water if all of the water has evaporated, and cook for another 2 to 3 minutes, without covering the pan. Add the spinach and cover the pan. Allow the spinach to wilt for 1 to 2 minutes. Plate the spinach and salmon, drizzle with $1/2$ teaspoon olive oil, and the remaining herb mixture, and serve.

HEALING PHASE SIDE DISHES

ASIAN STEAMED SPINACH WITH RAW SESAME SEEDS (V)

Serves 2   Prep and cooking time: 12 minutes

Any animal protein you choose—chicken breast, fish, or even a steak (on a special occasion)—goes with this mellow and subtle side dish.

    2 tablespoons Bragg Liquid Aminos
    11 ounces fresh baby spinach
    Handful of raw sesame seeds

In a medium saucepan, heat the Bragg Liquid Aminos over medium-high heat until they start to steam. Add the spinach and let the steaming liquid wilt it. Toss to distribute the heat evenly. Top with sesame seeds and serve.

WATERMELON MOZZARELLA COCKTAIL (F)

Serves 1   Prep time: 5 minutes

    10 (1-inch) watermelon cubes
    1 slice fresh buffalo mozzarella, cut up
    2 fresh basil leaves, chopped
    Pinch of Celtic salt

Place the watermelon, mozzarella, and basil in a bowl. Toss gently, then sprinkle with salt.

CANTALOUPE EXPRESS (F)

Serves 1   Prep time: 5 minutes

1/4 small cantaloupe, cubed

1 slice fresh buffalo mozzarella, cut up

2 small sprigs savory, chopped

2 small sprigs rosemary, chopped

Pinch of Celtic salt

Place the cantaloupe, mozzarella, and herbs in a bowl. Toss gently, then sprinkle with salt.

A HEARTY BOWL OF BUTTERY
BUCKWHEAT GROATS (G)

Serves 4 to 6   Prep and cooking time: 25 to 30 minutes

A staple of Asian and Eastern European cuisine, buckwheat groats are a healthful whole grain that's high in fiber, plant-based protein, pH, vitamins, minerals, and omega-3s. Other benefits of buckwheat are that it is gluten free and low in glycemic index. The glycemic index is a way to rank carbs according to how much they increase blood sugar after eating. High-index foods are generally rapidly digested and absorbed and result in large rises and falls in blood sugar levels. Low-index foods, because of their slow absorption, flatten out or eliminate sugar spikes and can help control appetite and therefore have benefits for weight control. While it has been cultivated in the United States since the colonial period, buckwheat hasn't gained the culinary following as a base or side dish enjoyed by popular grains like couscous, rice, quinoa, and bulgur. Yet its robust, nutty flavor, which absorbs and melds nicely with other foods, makes it an Acid Watcher–friendly side dish alternative. It is also delicious enough to be enjoyed by itself. All you need is some salt and organic butter for flavoring. Keep in mind that it is a finicky grain, not difficult to make but demanding precision. So follow these instructions closely.

2 cups filtered water

1 cup buckwheat groats

1 tablespoon organic butter

Dash of Celtic salt

In a medium pan, bring the water to a boil. Don't let too much water evaporate.

Add the buckwheat groats, butter, and salt. Reduce the heat to low, then cover and simmer for exactly 17 minutes, until the groats are soft (see Note).

Remove from the heat. Fluff the groats with a fork or a spatula, cover, and allow to rest for another 5 minutes before serving.

Note: Larger groats may require longer cooking time, up to 21 minutes. But don't overcook. Mushy buckwheat is not as satisfying in taste.

HEALING PHASE DESSERTS

ACID WATCHER HOT "CHOCOLATE"

Serves 1 to 2   Prep and cooking time: 10 minutes

This thick, hot, after-dinner drink has the goodness of traditional hot chocolate without the dietary complications that Acid Watchers need to avoid. You'll need a small double boiler and a whisk to make the mixture silky smooth. If you don't have a double boiler, you can improvise by placing a glass bowl over a pot of boiling water. Make sure the water doesn't come up to the bowl and that the bowl fits snugly over the pot so it doesn't wiggle around as you whisk. You wont miss chocolate once you get a taste of this hAWt ChAWcolate!

$1/3$ cup carob chips

1 cup coconut milk

1 tablespoon carob powder

$1/4$ teaspoon vanilla extract

$1/4$ teaspoon cinnamon

Bring water to a gentle boil in the bottom of a double boiler. Reduce the heat to medium-low.

Combine all of the ingredients in the top of the double boiler and continually whisk the mixture, as the carob chips melt, for 4 to 6 minutes. Serve immediately.

POACHED PEARS WITH CAROB
GANACHE AND PISTACHIOS (F)

Serves 2 to 4   Prep and cooking time: 45 minutes

This flavorful, light dessert can be made up to two days before serving. It is elegant enough to be served at a dinner party, but so easy you can whip it up in no time if a sweet tooth or chocolate withdrawal strikes during the Healing Phase. To make a ganache you will need a double boiler.

POACHED PEARS

   2 cups filtered water

   1 star anise

   5 whole cloves

   3-inch cinnamon stick

   1 inch fresh ginger, peeled

   1/2 cup dried Turkish apricots

   1/4 cup raisins

   2 Bosc pears, barely ripe

GANACHE

   1/2 cup carob chips

   1/3 cup almond milk

   1/4 teaspoon vanilla

   A dash of ground cinnamon

   1/4 cup unsalted pistachios, shelled

In a small pot, bring the filtered water, star anise, cloves, cinnamon stick, ginger, apricots, and raisins to a boil.

While the water is heating, prepare the pears by peeling them and cutting them in half, removing the core and stem with the tip of a paring knife.

Place the pears in the boiling liquid, reduce the heat, cover the pot, and simmer for 20 minutes. Remove from the heat and allow the pears to rest in the poaching liquid for another 20 minutes, then remove and refrigerate for at least 1/2 hour before serving. Discard the liquid and the aromatics and reserve the raisins and any apricots that have held their shape.

While the pears are simmering, prepare the ganache. Bring water to a boil in the bottom of a double boiler. Reduce to a simmer. Place the carob chips and almond milk in the top of the double boiler. Start whisking when the carob chips begin to melt. Add the vanilla and cinnamon. Continue whisking for 4 to 6 minutes, until a thick syrup forms. Remove from the heat and allow to cool.

In a small pan, toast the pistachios over high heat for 3 to 6 minutes. Stir frequently to prevent burning.

To serve, place each pear half in a bowl or on a dessert plate, drizzle with ganache, and top with pistachios and the poached apricots and raisins.

CHAPTER 11

The Maintenance Phase Meal Planner with Recipes

Congratulations on completing the Acid Watcher Healing Phase! The lifestyle changes you've committed to over the past 28 days have likely produced countless benefits within your body, hopefully improving your acid damage symptoms. By cutting out corrosive high-acid foods, you've put the brakes on inflammation and helped repair the esophageal tissue that's so essential to keeping acid reflux at bay. You should be experiencing relief from heartburn and/or throatburn, indigestion, bloating, and persistent food cravings. If you had throatburn reflux, your early-morning stuffiness and coughing that made you feel creaky and cranky has finally subsided. And the pounds—whether just a few or enough to necessitate a shopping spree for clothes a size smaller—melted off without the anguish of hunger or deprivation.

Graduating to the Maintenance Phase involves the strategic reintroduction of what are likely some of your favorite indulgences. If you've been yearning for the comfort of, let's say, a hearty stew, a flour-based dessert, a cup of coffee first thing in the morning, or the chilly ecstasy of a late-afternoon drink, you can now take a measured swill and still be a good Acid Watcher. The trick is to remember that the reintroduction of these foods has to be managed carefully, and you should listen to your body. If a food gives you that old feeling of reflux, it should be cut.

My advice is that you stick to the Maintenance Phase for at least two weeks after completing the Healing Phase. I designed it to be flexible enough for Acid Watchers to enjoy it and perhaps even make it their life's dietary journey. You don't have to do it, but I am betting you'll feel so good that you'll *want* to. Of course, like me or most other people, you may slip up now and again, indulging yourself in a binge of "Acid Watcher Dubious" food, but when the acid reflux makes an unwanted return, I predict that you'll be back on the wagon in no time.

In this second phase of the diet you should continue adhering to the same foundational principles as the Healing Phase: you will want to be smoke free, eat on time, continue to practice low-acid cooking techniques, and enjoy only **minimally processed food.**

A welcome difference in this phase is the loosening of the pH-based restrictions. The Maintenance Phase of the Acid Watcher Diet allows the inclusion of foods that measure pH 4, thus expanding the strict limits of the Rule of 5 that you practiced during the Healing Phase. It may seem like a slight modification, but it isn't. As I showed earlier in the book (see page 25), there is a substantial difference in acidity between foods that differ by a single point on the pH scale, so you'll find that with the inclusion of foods at pH 4 you'll have a broader list of options for delicious fruits, vegetables, dairy products, and grains that are excluded from many other pH-centered programs. If these aren't your trigger foods, you can expect to add the following items to your diet:

1. Red, yellow, and green bell peppers

2. Certain varieties of apples, grapes, and tropical fruit

3. Soft cheeses and cultured dairy products, including feta and cottage cheese

4. Yogurt, particularly the delicious and good-for-you Greek and kefir varieties. While other pH programs exclude yogurt and dairy from their eating plans, I believe that the health benefits of probiotics that prevail in certain types of dairy are too great to ignore. (Unless, of course, they happen to be your trigger foods.)

Although I don't recommend that the foods omitted from the Healing Phase be reintroduced simultaneously—too many of my patients

The Controversy Surrounding Probiotics

Although the science on probiotics is not conclusive, evidence suggests that they may profoundly affect brain-gut interactions ("microbiome-gut-brain-axis") and lessen the development of stress-induced disorders in both the upper and lower gastrointestinal tract. In addition, probiotics given to infants seem to reduce GERD-associated symptoms. (Further studies on the brain-gut axis are needed to explore other therapeutic benefits of probiotics.)

have reported the return of their symptoms if they rush to bring them all back at the same time—you can look forward to occasionally indulging in the following:

1. *Cooked* onion: Cooking onion appears to diminish its carminative effects. However, it does not seem to diminish its fructan effect. This means that if bloating is one of your symptoms, you should stay away from cooked onion.

2. *Cooked* garlic: Cooking garlic also appears to diminish its carminative effects. As with onions, the fructan effect doesn't go away in the process of cooking. So the same rule applies here: if bloating is one of your symptoms, stay away from cooked garlic. In its place, you can use leeks, a milder but satisfying vegetable from the onion family and a staple of French cuisine.

3. A *single cup* of coffee per day: Many people start their day with coffee, so if you feel that your symptoms have gone away at the end of the Healing Phase, go ahead and give your daily cup of joe a try. However, if your GERD symptoms return, the best thing for your health is to give it up.

4. Potato-based vodka: This spirit (Chopin, Long Island Vodka, or Spud brand) has a pH value of 5 and higher, so it is not nearly as

What Is a Leek?

A leek is a member of the onion and garlic family, a vegetable distinguished by its mellow, subtle flavor and versatility. You will instantly recognize the leek for its cylindrical shape, with the delicate, white and light green sheaths of leaves at the bottom, and the stringy dark green sprouts at the top, which can be used for flavoring but whose texture is not smooth enough to be enjoyed. A leek is an ideal partner to the potato, and is especially delicious when roasted, grilled, or used as an aromatic for fish and stocks. Remember to wash the leeks thoroughly as the grit tends to get stuck between layers.

acidic as grape-based wine. Again, the caveat with alcohol is that it is still a carminative, so limit your intake. And you should always have it on the rocks, not in a cocktail, which is most certainly laden with acidic pepsin stimulants.

5. **Corn-based vodka:** The same rules as for potato-based vodka apply here (Tito, Sobieski, or Balls brand).

6. **Dark chocolate:** If you don't have Barrett's esophagus, you can try having dark chocolate in small amounts (a 1-inch square no more than $1/4$ inch thick). Follow the same rule as you would in reintroducing coffee—if your symptoms return, chocolate must go.

THE MAINTENANCE PHASE EXTENDED FOODS LIST

You may notice that some of these "new foods" already appeared in the Healing Phase of the diet. What made those particular foods permissible during the initial phase of the diet was the fact that they were combined with much-higher-pH foods to create an overall safe pH. In the Maintenance Phase you'll be able to enjoy these foods alone, that is, without a more alkaline companion. Please keep in mind that pH levels can vary depending on the ripeness, freshness, or source of the product. Ripe fruits and vegetables tend to have a higher pH level than those that are not fully ripe.

pH 4 Raw Vegetables

Yellow bell pepper	4.8–5.44
Red bell pepper	4.8–5.24
Green bell pepper	4.8–5.89

pH 4 Raw and Dried Fruits

Apple (Red Delicious)	4.88
Kiwi	4.84
Mango	4.58
Figs	4.55
Apple (Golden Delicious)	4.5
Cherries	4.43
Raisins (dark)	4.41
Apple (Gala)	4.31
Prunes (dried)	4.27
Peach (yellow, ripe)	4.25
Pear (Forelle, ripe)	4.2
Blueberries	4.19
Pear (Bartlett, ripe)	4.15
Grapes (green seedless)	4.12

pH 4 Yogurt, Dairy, and Dairy Substitute Products

Cottage cheese	4.64
Butter (unsalted)	4.63
Feta cheese	4.6

Cream cheese (Philadelphia)	4.59
Yogurt (plain, Stonyfield)	4.43
Greek yogurt (plain, Fage)	4.34
Goat cheese	4.32
Greek yogurt (plain, Chobani)	4.31
Kefir	4.17
Almond yogurt (plain, Almond Dream)	4.67
Coconut milk, cultured (vanilla, So Delicious)	4.66
Soy yogurt (plain, Whole Soy & Co.)	4.64
Coconut milk, cultured (plain, So Delicious)	4.58
Soy yogurt (vanilla, Whole Soy & Co.)	4.44

pH 4 Condiments

Honey (manuka)	4.31
Agave nectar (light)	4.2

pH 4 Bread

Ezekiel 4:9 cinnamon raisin	4.64

The Honey Primer (What You Should Know About Manuka Versus Other Varieties)

All industrial food products are subject to questions regarding their nutrient composition, which takes such a hit during processing. Honey is no exception, so if you buy it at your local supermarket, chances are that it hasn't retained all of its anti-inflammatory, antibacterial, pro-digestive, medicinal properties for which it has been known since the earliest days of civilization. For that reason, the locally harvested honey sold at farmers' markets is a safer bet if you are buying honey not just as sweetener but as an edible healing agent. If it is locally produced, chances are that this honey wasn't processed at a factory on a distant continent and it will taste much, much better than its grocery store counterpart.

There is one type of honey from a distant continent that I do recommend for Acid Watchers. Manuka honey is harvested in New Zealand. It is derived from bees that pollinate the local manuka bush, and the product is distinguished by its unusually high content of antibacterial enzymes that aid in tissue healing and digestion. No one knows exactly why manuka flowers are so potent, but we know that the resulting honey stands far above the rest in its nutrient offering.

THE MAINTENANCE PHASE WEEKLY MEAL PLAN

For dieters who prefer to follow a weekly menu, here is an example of the one that has worked well for my patients. You could follow it for a week, two weeks, or longer if you like. But because some Acid Watchers may want to extend the Maintenance Phase for more than two mandatory weeks, I have given you more options to choose from and an additional weekly plan of menus to use as an example. Keep in mind that you are free to continue using recipes from the Healing Phase, except now you can add the permitted ingredients measuring above pH 4.

MAINTENANCE PHASE WEEK 1 MEAL PLAN

	DAY 1	DAY 2	DAY 3	DAY 4	DAY 5	DAY 6	DAY 7
Breakfast 7–9 a.m.	F Pineapple Express Smoothie (p. 203)	E/D Yogurt with Raisins and Almonds (p. 203)	G Acid Watcher Blueberry Crepes (p. 159)	F Dr. Aviv's Berry Smoothie Blast (p. 158)	E/D Spinach Omelet (p. 161)	G Pear Oatmeal (p. 162)	V Green Juice (p. 158)
Morning Mini-Meal 10–11 a.m.	V Guac Tapenade Toast (p. 164)	F Fresh fruit (8 ounces)	V Raw veggies	E/D Hard-boiled egg	F Fresh fruit (8 ounces)	E/D Mozzarella Herb Toast (p. 164)	N Toast with almond butter and honey
Lunch 12:30–2:00 p.m.	AP Mexican Shrimp Salad with Avocado, Black Beans, and Cilantro (p. 179)	V High-Fiber Salad (p. 166)	AP Pesto Chicken Sandwich (p. 167)	V Kale Wrap with Guac Tapenade (p. 168)	V Vegetable Pasta Salad (p. 169)	AP Colorful Chicken Salad (p. 170)	AP Stuffed Baked Salmon with Sweet Potato (p. 213)
Afternoon Mini-Meal 3–4 p.m.	N/F Dr. Aviv's Power Bar (p. 165)	N Assorted tree nuts	F Fresh fruit (6–7 ounces)	N/F Almond butter and banana	N Assorted tree nuts	F Fresh fruit (5–6 ounces)	F Peach Blossom Smoothie (p. 202)
Dinner 6–7:30 p.m.	V Kale "Cobb" Salad (p. 227)	AP Miso-Agave-Glazed Halibut with Sesame Bok Choy (p. 174)	V Brussels Sprout Salad with Pecans, Raisins, and Apple (p. 228)	AP Turkey Burger with Arugula-Ginger Salad (p. 175)	AP Broiled Herbed Salmon with Steamed Spinach (p. 171)	V Papaya Salad (p. 177)	V Puréed Butternut Squash Soup with Seared Mushrooms and Herbs (p. 184)

MAINTENANCE PHASE WEEK 2 MEAL PLAN

	DAY 1	DAY 2	DAY 3	DAY 4	DAY 5	DAY 6	DAY 7
Breakfast 7–9 a.m.	F Peach Cobbler Smoothie (p. 205)	G Mango Oatmeal "Brûlée" (p. 205)	F Papaya Chill Smoothie (p. 202)	F Tropic Thunder Smoothie (p. 203)	E/D Healthy Fruit-Flavored Yogurt #1 or #2 (p. 204)	E/D Goat Cheese and Spinach Frittata (p. 207)	AP Savory Continental Breakfast Special (p. 206)
Morning Mini-Meal 10–11 a.m.	V Raw veggies	N Toast with almond butter and honey	G A Hearty Bowl of Buttery Buckwheat Groats (p. 188)	N Assorted tree nuts, 1 T carob chips, 1 Turkish dried apricot	V Lima Bean "Faux" Hummus (p. 211)	F Fresh fruit (8 ounces)	F Fresh fruit (8 ounces)
Lunch 12:30–2:00 p.m.	G Wild Mushroom Barley Soup (p. 218)	V Brussels Sprout Salad with Pecans, Raisins, and Apple (p. 228)	V Kale "Cobb" Salad (p. 227)	AP Pesto Chicken Sandwich (p. 167)	V Smooth and Crunchy Kale Salad (p. 215)	V Sautéed Portobello and Sweet Pepper Sandwich with Basil-Avocado Crema (p. 214)	V Roasted and Fresh Vegetable GAWzpacho (p. 216)
Afternoon Mini-Meal 3–4 p.m.	V Olive-Artichoke Pâté (p. 210)	F Fresh fruit (8 ounces)	E/D Apple-Beet Tapenade (p. 209)	V Raw veggies	V Raw veggies	N Assorted tree nuts	N/F Dr. Aviv's Power Bar (p. 165)
Dinner 6–7:30 p.m.	AP Fresh Fish en Papillote with Potatoes, Olives, and Leeks (p. 224)	AP Fish and Chips (p. 176) with Sauté of Fennel, Red Cabbage, and Swiss Chard (p. 226)	AP Herb Chicken (p. 181) with Asian Steamed Spinach with Raw Sesame Seeds (p. 187)	V Puréed Butternut Squash Soup with Seared Mushrooms and Herbs (p. 184)	AP Poached Salmon with Creamy Ginger-Dill Sauce (p. 221)	AP Cauliflower "Paella" with Shrimp and Chicken (p. 220)	AP Lean and Mean Cottage Pie (p. 222)

Recipes for the Maintenance Phase

MAINTENANCE PHASE BREAKFAST RECIPES

PEACH BLOSSOM SMOOTHIE (F)

Serves 1   Prep time: 5 minutes

1 peach, halved and pitted

1 mango, peeled and cubed

1 small banana

1 tablespoon plain yogurt

$1/2$ teaspoon vanilla extract (optional)

Handful of ice

Combine all of the ingredients in a blender and blend until smooth. Pour into a glass and enjoy.

PAPAYA CHILL SMOOTHIE (F)

Serves 1   Prep time: 5 to 10 minutes

1 cup papaya chunks

2 tablespoons plain regular yogurt

$1/2$ banana

$1/2$ cup ice

Combine all of the ingredients in a blender and blend until smooth. Pour into a glass and enjoy.

PINEAPPLE EXPRESS SMOOTHIE (F)
Serves 1   Prep time: 5 to 10 minutes

$1/2$ cup pineapple chunks (see Note)
$1/2$ cup papaya chunks
$1/2$ banana
$1/3$ cup soy milk
Handful of ice

Combine all of the ingredients in a blender and blend until smooth. Pour into a glass and enjoy.

Note: Pineapple is acidic but when mixed with other ingredients in proper proportion, as in this smoothie, the acidity is neutralized.

TROPIC THUNDER SMOOTHIE (F)
Serves 1   Prep time: 5 to 10 minutes

1 small mango, peeled and cubed
$1/2$ cup papaya chunks
3 to 4 fresh lychees, peeled, pitted, and halved
$1/2$ dragon fruit, peeled and halved
$1/2$ banana
1 tablespoon yogurt
$1/2$ cup ice

Combine all of the ingredients in a blender and blend until smooth. Pour into a glass and enjoy.

YOGURT WITH RAISINS AND ALMONDS (D)
Serves 2   Prep time: 5 minutes

3 tablespoons plain yogurt
$1/2$ banana
2 teaspoons raisins

1 teaspoon ground raw almonds or walnuts

Honey, to taste

Mix together the yogurt, banana, raisins, and nuts. Drizzle with honey and serve.

HEALTHY FRUIT-FLAVORED YOGURT #1 (F)

Serves 2   Prep time: 5 minutes

$1/2$ cup frozen strawberries

$1/2$ cup frozen blueberries

$1/2$ cup unsweetened almond milk

$1/2$ cup plain kefir

1 teaspoon honey

Combine all of the ingredients in a blender and blend until smooth. Pour into a glass and enjoy.

HEALTHY FRUIT-FLAVORED YOGURT #2 (F)

Serves 2   Prep time: 5 minutes

1 cup frozen cherries

1 cup diced ripe pear

1 cup plain kefir

$1/2$ cup full-fat Greek yogurt

$1/4$ cup slivered almonds, blanched hazelnuts, or walnuts

1 teaspoon honey

Place the cherries, pear, kefir, and yogurt in a blender and pulse until smooth. Pour into a glass or a bowl. Top with the nuts, drizzle with honey, and serve.

PEACH COBBLER SMOOTHIE (G)
Serves 2   Prep time: 5 minutes

1 cup frozen peaches
2/3 cup cooked buckwheat groats (see page 188)
1/4 teaspoon vanilla extract
1/4 teaspoon baking spice
1/2 teaspoon ground cinnamon
2 teaspoons honey
2 cups plain kefir

Combine all of the ingredients in a blender and blend until smooth. Pour into a glass and enjoy.

MANGO OATMEAL "BRÛLÉE" (G)
Serves 2
Prep and cooking time: 30 minutes, plus 20 minutes for soaking the oats

This luxurious but easy-to-prepare breakfast will get you out of bed faster than coffee. The almond milk in which the oatmeal is slowly simmered neutralizes the acidity of the mango, a touch of cinnamon gives it the richness of a dessert, and the nuts add the crunch and a small dose of healthy fats that will keep you away from unhealthy snacks throughout the morning. Don't use instant oatmeal—it is overprocessed and therefore more acidic than the whole-grain version. Soaking the oatmeal overnight, especially if you are using steel-cut oats, will give your oatmeal a soufflé consistency. But if you don't want to think about your breakfast the night before, regular rolled oats or Irish oatmeal will do just as well. A 20-minute soak prior to cooking will produce rewarding results.

1/2 cup steel-cut oats, rolled oats, or Irish oats, soaked in 1 cup
    filtered water
Dash of Celtic salt

1 medium ripe Haitian mango, peeled and cubed

$1/2$ cup filtered water

$1/2$ cup unsweetened, full-fat almond milk

$1/2$ teaspoon ground cinnamon

2 tablespoons toasted and chopped walnuts or slivered, toasted almonds

Combine the soaked oats, salt, mango, filtered water, and almond milk in a nonstick pan and bring to a boil. Reduce the heat to low, cover the pan tightly, and simmer for 5 to 7 minutes, stirring with a wooden spoon once or twice to prevent sticking. The liquids should be absorbed and the oatmeal gooey.

Remove from the heat and keep the pan covered for 20 minutes, allowing all the flavors to meld.

Serve the oatmeal at room temperature, topped with cinnamon and nuts.

SAVORY CONTINENTAL
BREAKFAST SPECIAL (AP)
Serves 1   Prep time: 15 minutes

This is a breakfast for champions—high in flavor and variety, low in sugar and acid, minimal kitchen skills required. Reserve the remaining asparagus for your lunch or dinner side dish.

1 large egg, soft- or hard-boiled

3 blanched asparagus spears (can be made in advance; see Note)

1 slice toasted whole-grain or spelt-grain bread

$1/4$ Hass avocado, pitted, scooped, and mashed with a dash of Celtic salt

2 ounces smoked salmon

4 slices Kirby, Persian, or seedless English cucumber

To make a soft-boiled egg, place the egg in a small pan, cover with water, and bring to a boil. Reduce the heat, cover the pan, and simmer for 4 minutes. Remove the egg from the water with a slotted spoon and plunge immediately into a bowl of ice water to stop the cooking and for easy peeling. To make a hard-boiled egg, follow the same directions but simmer the egg for 7 minutes.

Bring a pot of salted water to a boil. While the water is heating, prepare the asparagus by washing it thoroughly and trimming the ends. The best way to trim the asparagus is by snapping the stalk while holding it gently with your fingers at both ends. It will break naturally precisely at the point where the soft part ends and the fibrous, tough part begins. Reserve and freeze the fibrous parts of asparagus for vegetable or chicken broth.

Blanch the asparagus for 7 minutes, until crisp tender (see instructions for blanching on page 135).

Spread the avocado on the toast. Top with salmon and cucumber slices. Arrange the toast, egg, and asparagus stalks on a plate and serve immediately.

Note: It is silly to make three spears of asparagus, so you may just as well make a bunch and add them to your meals throughout the day.

GOAT CHEESE AND SPINACH FRITTATA (AP)
Serves 2 to 4   Prep and cooking time: 25 minutes

A frittata is an Italian-style omelet that is cooked on the stovetop halfway through and finished in the oven. It sounds complicated, but I assure you that you don't have to be a ninja in the kitchen to master the process. To make the frittata, all you will need besides the ingredients and these instructions is a 9-inch nonstick pan. A universal crowd pleaser, a frittata can be served hot or at room temperature. With a side of a salad and an Acid Watcher–friendly fruit or dessert, it is a perfect choice for a healthy brunch. With plenty of protein and healthy fats, it should keep you satiated for hours.

4 large eggs

1 to 2 tablespoons filtered water

Dash of Celtic salt

$1/4$ cup crumbled goat cheese

$1/2$ ripe Hass avocado, pitted, scooped, and roughly chopped

1 tablespoon organic butter

1 cup fresh baby spinach

$1/4$ cup shredded Parmesan cheese

Preheat the oven to 375°F.

In a medium bowl, whisk the eggs with the filtered water and the salt. Fold in the goat cheese and avocado.

Melt the butter in a heated pan. Add the spinach. Stir with a wooden spatula until the leaves are wilted. Make sure they are spread out evenly at the bottom of the pan.

Slowly pour the egg mixture over the spinach and allow to set over medium-high heat for about 5 minutes, until the sides of the frittata begin to turn crispy. Do not stir.

Remove from the heat and sprinkle the Parmesan on top of the frittata. Bake for 5 minutes.

Preheat the broiler to 400°F. and cook for 2 to 3 minutes more, until the Parmesan is melted and the center of the frittata is cooked through but still jiggly. Remove from the oven and allow to rest for 3 minutes before serving.

MAINTENANCE PHASE MINI-MEALS

APPLE-BEET TAPENADE (AP)
Serves 4 to 6
Prep and cooking time: 10 to 15 minutes, plus 2 hours for
roasting and cooling the beets

Even though we think of tapenade as a mix of olives, garlic, capers, and infinite other variations of Mediterranean-style ingredients, there is no reason to restrict one's options when it comes to putting together creative open sandwiches. The medley of beets, apples, nuts, and goat cheese is a refreshing, colorful alternative that can be enjoyed as a spread on whole-grain toast, as a dip, or as a small side salad. Roast the beets in advance, preferably overnight so they can absorb all the flavors. Goat cheese makes this tapenade especially creamy, and it is better for you than cow's milk–based cream cheeses.

3 medium beets, peeled
$1/4$ teaspoon ground fennel
$1/4$ teaspoon ground cumin
$1/4$ teaspoon ground coriander
$1/4$ cup filtered water
Celtic salt, to taste
$1/3$ cup walnuts
2 ounces goat cheese
$1/4$ teaspoon ground sumac
1 tablespoon fresh cilantro leaves
$1/2$ Golden Delicious apple, cored and peeled

Preheat the oven to 400°F.

Combine the beets, fennel, cumin, coriander, filtered water, and salt to taste in a small casserole dish, cover, and roast for 1 hour, turning the beets every 20 minutes to make sure they roast evenly. Remove from the oven when done, and allow the beets to come to room temperature.

In a food processor, pulse the walnuts, goat cheese, sumac, and cilantro for 30 to 60 seconds, until the mixture reaches an oatmeal-like consistency.

In a large bowl, grate the beets and the apple. Add the walnut-and-goat-cheese mixture and combine with a spoon. Add salt to taste. Allow the tapenade to rest for 1 hour before serving to meld the flavors.

OLIVE-ARTICHOKE PÂTÉ (V)

Serves 12   Prep and cooking time: 25 to 35 minutes

This Acid Watcher–friendly variation on the popular but garlic-and-lemon-heavy spinach and artichoke dip is a perfect party starter or snack to be enjoyed on whole-grain toast or as a dip with crudités.

    1 teaspoon olive oil
    1 cup fresh baby spinach
    1 cup fresh baby arugula
    1 tablespoon vegetable broth or filtered water
    Celtic salt, to taste
    1 cup frozen artichoke hearts, thawed
    4 large green olives, pitted
    4 ounces goat cheese
    1/2 cup plain kefir
    1/4 cup shredded white Cheddar cheese
    1/4 cup shredded Parmesan cheese

Preheat the oven to 400°F.

In a preheated nonstick pan, heat the oil and sauté the spinach and arugula for 3 to 4 minutes, until the leaves are wilted. Loosen them with broth or water if needed to prevent sticking. Flavor with a sprinkle of salt.

In a food processor, pulse the artichoke hearts, olives, and goat cheese under a steady stream of kefir.

Place the mixture with the spinach and arugula in a deep casserole dish and fold in the Cheddar cheese. Even out the mixture with a spatula and sprinkle with the Parmesan. Bake for 22 to 25 minutes, until the cheeses have melted and the mixture is bubbly.

Preheat the broiler and broil for 2 minutes more, until the outer edges of the dip turn crispy brown. Serve warm or at room temperature.

LIMA BEAN "FAUX" HUMMUS (V)
Serves 10 to 12
Prep and cooking time: 25 minutes, plus more for cooling

For Acid Watchers desperate for a taste of hummus, this lima bean condiment provides a tasty alternative. The Middle Eastern spice mix za'atar gives it an authentic flavor. This faux hummus is especially satisfying with black olives and a homemade roasted bell pepper on top, which add texture, brininess, and a splash of color to every bite.

- 2 red, yellow, or orange bell peppers
- 1 tablespoon olive oil
- 1 medium leek, thoroughly washed, chopped (white part only)
- 1 cup frozen baby lima beans, thawed
- $1/4$ teaspoon ground sumac
- 1 teaspoon za'atar
- 1 cup vegetable broth
- 1 tablespoon finely chopped fresh parsley leaves
- $1/4$ cup pitted black olives, drained (optional)

Preheat the oven to 400°F. Wash the peppers and place them on a baking sheet lined with parchment paper. Roast for 30 minutes, turning the peppers over with tongs halfway through the roasting process. Remove the baking sheet from the oven. When the peppers are cool enough to handle, remove the stems, ribs, seeds, and skin. Slice into thin strips.

While the peppers are roasting and cooling, prepare the hummus. In a preheated nonstick pan, heat the oil and sauté the leek for about 2 minutes, until soft. Add the lima beans, sumac, and za'atar and reduce to a simmer. Cook, stirring constantly, for 15 to 20 minutes, loosening the mixture with the broth $1/3$ cup at a time, until all of the liquid is absorbed. Fold in the parsley.

Allow the mixture to come to room temperature and pulse in a food processor until it reaches the degree of smoothness you desire. Serve immediately, topped with olives (if using) and sliced roasted bell peppers.

MAINTENANCE PHASE LUNCH RECIPES

STUFFED BAKED SALMON WITH
SWEET POTATO (AP)

Serves 1   Prep and cooking time: 25 minutes

Serve this perfect weekday lunch or dinner with a side of lightly steamed kale.

> 2 to 3 teaspoons olive oil
>
> 1/2 medium sweet potato, sliced into circles
>
> Celtic salt, to taste
>
> 5 to 6 ounces salmon fillet, skin on
>
> 2 to 3 tablespoons finely chopped leek (white part only)
>
> 3 to 4 teaspoons Bragg Liquid Aminos
>
> 2 lemon slices
>
> 2 teaspoons chopped fresh rosemary

Preheat the oven to 450°F. Line a small baking sheet with foil and brush it with the oil. Spread the sweet potato circles around the edges of the pan and sprinkle with salt.

Place the salmon fillet on a cutting board, skin side down. Cut across the fillet lengthwise, almost splitting it in half as you would a hot dog bun. Sprinkle with salt all around.

In a small bowl, combine the leek and 3 teaspoons of the Bragg Liquid Aminos. Stuff the filling into the salmon fillet. Close and top with the lemon slices. Sprinkle the rosemary on top.

Bake for about 15 minutes, until the fish and the potato are cooked, turning the potato slices over about halfway through the cooking process. You do not need to flip the fish over.

Remove the fish and potato slices from the oven, sprinkle the fish with more Bragg Liquid Aminos, and serve immediately.

SAUTÉED PORTOBELLO AND SWEET PEPPER SANDWICH WITH BASIL-AVOCADO CREMA (V)

Serves 2   Prep and cooking time: 15 minutes

This vegetarian sandwich makes for a quick, delicious, and filling lunch or a light supper on a hot summer day. It looks, sounds, and tastes gourmet but requires minimal effort to make.

> 1 portobello mushroom (approximately $2^1/2$ ounces), stem removed, cleaned with a wet paper towel
>
> 1 to 2 tablespoons olive oil
>
> $1/4$ teaspoon dried oregano
>
> $1/4$ teaspoon dried marjoram
>
> $1/4$ teaspoon dried thyme
>
> Celtic salt, to taste
>
> 1 medium red or orange bell pepper, cored and cut into strips
>
> 4 slices sprouted wheat bread
>
> 1 tablespoon avocado or olive oil
>
> $1/2$ ripe Hass avocado, pitted and scooped
>
> 3 fresh basil leaves
>
> 1 tablespoon plain Greek yogurt
>
> 1 teaspoon ground sumac

Using a paring knife, scrape the gills from the underside of the portobello cap and slice the cap into thick slivers. You should have 7 to 8 slices. Heat 1 tablespoon of the olive oil in a nonstick pan over a medium flame for 30 seconds. Add the portobello slices in a single layer and sauté for 2 to 3 minutes on each side. Sprinkle with water, if needed, to prevent burning. Add the oregano, marjoram, thyme, and salt and cook for a minute more. Remove from the heat and place the portobello slices in a bowl.

Add the remaining 1 tablespoon olive oil and the bell pepper strips to the pan and sauté for 2 to 3 minutes, until the strips start to soften. Place in the bowl with the portobello slices.

Toast the bread.

While the bread is toasting, place the avocado (or olive) oil, avocado, basil, yogurt, and sumac in a food processor and pulse until the mixture is creamy.

Prepare the sandwiches by spreading the avocado crema on two of the toast slices. Top them with the portobello and bell pepper slices and the other two slices of bread. Serve immediately.

SMOOTH AND CRUNCHY KALE SALAD (V)
Serves 2 to 4   Prep time: 20 minutes

Kale is a vegetable that likes a good massage. If you've ever had a fresh kale salad that seemed fibrous and tough, I can tell you that it wasn't properly massaged. Massaging kale for a couple of minutes will coax the greatest textures and flavors from this generous plant. Red cabbage and carrots don't mind a massage either, and together with kale they form a trio as beautiful in appearance as it is potent in nutrients and flavor. All you have to do is put the three in a sieve over a bowl, sprinkle generously with salt, wait for 10 minutes, and massage until the vegetables start releasing moisture, becoming soft and succulent. Most grocery stores sell shredded red cabbage and carrots, which I recommend you buy for this salad. It will save you a lot of prep time.

- 6 ounces Tuscan kale (or any other kale)
- 3 ounces shredded red cabbage
- 2 ounces shredded carrot
- Dash of Celtic salt
- 1/4 cup sunflower seeds
- 1/3 cup feta cheese, preferably Bulgarian but Greek will do, cubed or crumbled
- 1/2 teaspoon ground sumac
- 2 teaspoons olive oil
- 1 ripe Hass avocado, pitted, scooped, and cubed

Toss the kale, cabbage, and carrot in a large sieve. Sprinkle generously with salt and let rest for 10 minutes.

While the vegetables are resting, toast the sunflower seeds in a hot, dry pan for about 3 minutes, until the seeds release their aroma and start browning. Don't walk away; seeds can burn quickly. Place the seeds into a salad bowl.

Massage the vegetables with your fingers, squeezing out as much water as you can. The volume of the vegetables should be reduced by approximately one third.

Dry the vegetables with a paper towel and transfer them to the salad bowl with sunflower seeds. Add the feta cheese, sumac, olive oil, and salt to taste. Toss.

Divide into bowls, top with avocado cubes, and serve immediately.

ROASTED AND FRESH VEGETABLE GAWZPACHO (V)
Serves 4 to 6
Prep and cooking time: 1 hour 15 minutes, plus cooling time

Gazpacho is a cold tomato-and-cucumber-based soup indigenous to Spanish cuisine, with countless variations that have developed in family and restaurant kitchens over generations. While tomatoes are off-limits to Acid Watchers during the Healing Phase, they can be served—if neutralized by a seedless cucumber—in the Maintenance Phase. In this recipe we use grape tomatoes, which are naturally less acidic and are further neutralized by fresh cucumbers, another gazpacho ingredient. The onion—used raw in some versions of gazpacho—is cooked at high temperature for the Maintenance Phase. The juice of tomatoes (often canned) used as the base for gazpacho is replaced with homemade or organic vegetable broth. But you won't miss it—the smokiness of roasted peppers, the flavor of the grape tomatoes, and the garden brightness of tarragon are as potent and refreshing as a summer day. A sprinkle of sumac gives the soup a hint of tartness. If you prefer your soups on the smoother, less chunky side, you can thin the gazpacho by running it through a strainer or a soup mill. For fancier presentation, dress it up with a gremolata (finely chopped ingredients served on top of the soup) of cubed avocado and crabmeat lumps, or a dollop of Greek yogurt.

> 6 ounces grape tomatoes
>
> 4 bell peppers (red, yellow, green, or a combination)
>
> 4 tablespoons olive oil
>
> 2 to 4 celery stalks
>
> $1/2$ Vidalia onion, roughly chopped
>
> Fresh tarragon leaves, from 10 sprigs
>
> 2 teaspoons Celtic salt
>
> 2 cups homemade or organic vegetable broth, plus more to sauté the vegetables
>
> 2 teaspoons sumac
>
> 4 Kirby or Persian cucumbers (or 1 English cucumber), finely grated
>
> $1/2$ Hass avocado, pitted and scooped (optional)
>
> 1 ounce fresh crabmeat (optional)
>
> 4 to 6 teaspoons plain Greek yogurt (optional)

Preheat the oven to 400°F. Lay out the tomatoes and bell peppers separately on two baking sheets lined with parchment paper or foil.

Roast the tomatoes for 20 minutes, turning them over on the baking sheet once they start blistering and releasing their juices, about 10 minutes into roasting.

Roast the bell peppers on the bottom rack for 50 to 60 minutes, turning over with plastic tongs every 20 minutes to make sure they are charred evenly. (Be careful not to puncture the skin of the bell peppers with tongs when turning.)

While the tomatoes and bell peppers are roasting, in a sauté pan, heat 2 tablespoons of the oil over medium-high heat. Sauté the celery, onion, tarragon, and 1 teaspoon of the salt for 20 minutes, stirring frequently to prevent sticking and burning. Drizzle broth into the pan to loosen the vegetables. The longer they sauté and the more broth they absorb, the more flavorful they will become.

Let the tomatoes and bell peppers cool to room temperature after roasting. (For optimal results with the bell peppers, place them in a sealed paper bag to cool. The skin will be easier to peel.)

Prepare the bell peppers after they have cooled by peeling the skin with your hands, removing the seeds and stems. Reserve the peeled bell peppers, along with their liquids, in a bowl with the tomatoes and their juices.

When the tomatoes, bell peppers, and sautéed vegetables are all at room temperature, place them in a food processor and pulse while pouring, in a stream, the remaining 2 tablespoons oil and 2 cups broth until the mixture is soupy. Pour into a sealed container and refrigerate for at least 4 hours before serving.

After the gazpacho has been chilled, put the finishing touches on it by adding salt to taste and stirring in the sumac and cucumbers. (If you want a smoother, thinner gazpacho, run it through a strainer or a food mill *before* adding the cucumbers.)

Serve in a bowl, with a topping of chopped avocado, crabmeat, and a dollop of Greek yogurt if desired.

WILD MUSHROOM BARLEY SOUP (G)
Serves 12 to 16
Prep and cooking time: 1 hour 45 minutes

The ultimate in winter comfort food, this soup is a full meal that gets tastier a day or two after it is cooked. And you can freeze the leftovers for up to a month! Wild mushrooms are the best option for this soup, giving it an inviting woodsy aroma and meaty texture. Fiber-full barley thickens the vegetable-infused broth, making the soup extra chewy. Homemade Chicken Broth (page 229) is the best cooking liquid for this soup, but if you want to make this dish vegan, you can use Vegetable Stock instead (page 231). To make the soup even more healthful and colorful, add a handful of baby spinach or kale when you reheat individual servings. Just keep heating the soup until the greens wilt and serve while piping hot. A dollop of Greek yogurt will make it even more slurp-worthy.

$2^1/2$ ounces dried mushrooms (porcini, shiitake, or a combination)

2 tablespoons olive oil

2 medium onions, finely chopped

2 celery stalks, finely chopped

2 medium carrots, grated

1 garlic clove, finely chopped

1 to 3 teaspoons Celtic salt

$3^1/2$ ounces fresh shiitake mushrooms, stems removed and
  reserved for vegetable broth

2 dried bay leaves

$1/4$ teaspoon dried rosemary

$1/4$ teaspoon dried thyme

$1/4$ teaspoon dried dill

1 teaspoon dried parsley

$2/3$ cup pearl barley

2 cups mushroom soaking liquid

1 quart chicken or vegetable broth

Soak the dried mushrooms in a bowl filled with 2 cups water for at least 4 hours or overnight.

Drain the rehydrated mushrooms, reserving the soaking liquid. Chop the mushrooms into small bite-size pieces, as they will expand during cooking.

In a 5-quart pot with a nonstick bottom, heat the oil over medium heat. Sauté the onions, celery, carrots, garlic, and 1 teaspoon of the salt for 15 to 20 minutes, stirring frequently to prevent sticking or burning, until the vegetables are soft and golden brown. Sprinkle with filtered water or broth to loosen the mixture if needed.

Add the fresh shiitake mushrooms and salt to taste and cook for 5 to 7 minutes, until the mushrooms are softened and browned.

Add the bay leaves, rosemary, thyme, dill, parsley, barley, mushroom soaking liquid, broth, and salt to taste, and bring to a high boil. Reduce to a simmer, cover the pot, and cook for 1 hour more, until the barley is soft.

When the soup has cooled somewhat, add salt to taste—this soup takes a lot of salt, so don't be alarmed if it keeps asking for more.

MAINTENANCE PHASE DINNER RECIPES

CAULIFLOWER "PAELLA" WITH
SHRIMP AND CHICKEN (AP)
Serves 2 to 4   Prep and cooking time: 25 minutes

This filling main course replaces rice with raw cauliflower, which is pulsed in a food processor to grainlike consistency and lightly sautéed on the stovetop in a little bit of olive oil and saffron. Chicken breast chunks, shrimp, and peas add a layer of texture, with herbs and spices adding a flash of aroma. Tastes great hot or cold!

> 2 boneless, skinless chicken breasts, cut into bite-size chunks
> 3 tablespoons olive oil
> 1 teaspoon Celtic salt, plus more to taste
> $1/4$ teaspoon fennel seeds
> $1/4$ teaspoon dried basil
> $1/2$ pound fresh shrimp (defrosted if frozen), preferably large or jumbo, shelled and deveined
> Pinch of saffron
> $1/2$ large head cauliflower, cored and separated into florets
> $3/4$ cup blanched petite peas, fresh or frozen (defrosted and drained)
> $1/4$ cup fresh cilantro leaves
> $1/4$ cup finely chopped fresh flat-leaf parsley leaves
> $1/2$ teaspoon ground sumac (optional)

Preheat the oven to 400°F. Line a baking sheet with foil. Toss the chicken chunks with 1 teaspoon of the oil, 1 teaspoon salt, and the fennel seeds and basil and spread on the baking sheet in a single layer. Roast for 10 minutes, flipping the chicken chunks over once halfway through the roasting process. Remove from the oven immediately to prevent overcooking.

Toss the shrimp with 1 tablespoon of the oil and salt to taste, and spread on a separate baking sheet lined with foil or parchment paper.

Roast for 6 minutes. Remove from the oven immediately to prevent over-cooking.

In a sauté pan, heat the remaining 1 tablespoon oil, $1/4$ cup water, and the saffron over medium-high heat. Place the cauliflower florets in a food processor and pulse until they are reduced to a grainy mass. Make sure not to overdo it, as the cauliflower can become too watery. When the oil in the pan begins to sizzle, add the cauliflower and sauté for 7 minutes. You want the cauliflower to attain a toasted and crunchy texture. The saffron threads will give the cauliflower beautiful rivulets of yellow.

Add the chicken, shrimp, peas, cilantro, and parsley and stir. Reduce the heat to low, cover the pan, and allow the paella to simmer for about 1 minute to allow the flavors to meld. Sprinkle with sumac (if using) and serve.

POACHED SALMON WITH CREAMY GINGER-DILL SAUCE (AP)
Serves 1 or 2, depending on how many fillets are poached
Prep and cooking time: 20 minutes

This versatile dish can be served for dinner with leftovers or reserved for a snack or lunch the next day. When accompanied by a simple salad, brown rice, or quinoa, the salmon fillet with creamy ginger-dill sauce makes for a complete and filling meal. Cooking it is easy, and its by-products are delicious. For example, you can use the poaching liquid (which yields about 2 cups) instead of water to cook 1 cup brown rice or quinoa. The poaching liquid will infuse grains with complex and inviting aromas. The leftover ginger-dill sauce can be used to dress tuna fish or leftover chicken for an open sandwich filling that you can have for breakfast, lunch, or a snack the next day.

> 3 cups homemade or organic vegetable broth
> $1/2$ cup fresh dill, including stems
> $1/2$ cup fresh cilantro, including stems
> 2 1-inch pieces fresh ginger, peeled
> 1 tablespoon Bragg Liquid Aminos

1 dried bay leaf

1 or 2 (6-ounce) salmon fillets, skinned

2 ounces soft tofu

1 Kirby or Persian cucumber, chopped roughly

$1/2$ apple, cored, peeled, and quartered (any apple other than a
green)

2 tablespoons olive oil

Dash of Celtic salt

1 tablespoon white miso

In a shallow nonstick pan, combine the broth, dill, cilantro, 1 piece of the ginger, Bragg Liquid Aminos, and bay leaf and bring to a boil.

Place the salmon fillets in the pan, reduce the heat to low, cover, and simmer for 8 to 10 minutes, until the fillets turn pale pink and are cooked all the way through. Remove to a plate or storage container to prevent overcooking. Drain and reserve the cooking liquid for another use. Discard the solids.

While the salmon is poaching, make the sauce by combining the tofu, cucumber, apple, oil, salt, miso, and the remaining piece of ginger in a food processor and pulsing until the consistency is smooth and creamy.

Serve the salmon cold or at room temperature, topped with the ginger-dill sauce.

LEAN AND MEAN COTTAGE PIE (AP)
Serves 4 to 6   Prep and cooking time: 45 to 50 minutes

Just because you are an Acid Watcher doesn't mean you should deprive yourself of an occasional comfort food such as an unbeatable combination of meat and potatoes. Shepherd's pie made of lamb and potatoes has kept the Irish people cozy and warm since time immemorial, and in England, the classic cottage pie made of ground beef and potatoes has inoculated many against the assault of the island's persistent frigid temperatures. Our cottage pie has all the deliciousness of the traditional dish without the acidic or fatty ingredients. We use ground turkey instead of red meat, and reduce the dairy component by using vegetable broth in place of whole milk to whip up the potatoes. If dairy is your trigger food, you can make the dish completely dairy free by using olive oil instead of butter.

> 1 teaspoon Celtic salt, plus more to taste
>
> 8 medium Yukon Gold potatoes, peeled and quartered
>
> 1 tablespoon olive oil
>
> 2 medium leeks (white parts only), thoroughly washed and finely chopped
>
> 1 medium carrot, grated
>
> $1^1/3$ cups homemade or organic vegetable broth
>
> 1 pound ground turkey (a mix of dark and white meat)
>
> 3 tablespoons Bragg Liquid Aminos
>
> $1/4$ cup chopped fresh dill, plus more for garnish
>
> 1 teaspoon dried thyme
>
> 1 teaspoon asafetida
>
> 1 tablespoon whole-wheat flour
>
> 2 tablespoons organic butter (replace with olive oil for a dairy-free option)

In a pot of generously salted water, bring the potatoes to a boil. Reduce the heat to low, cover, and simmer for 15 to 20 minutes, until the potatoes are cooked through but not mushy.

While the potatoes are cooking, in a medium sauté pan, heat the oil and sauté the leeks and carrot over medium heat for about 12 minutes, until the carrot is soft. Drizzle approximately $1/3$ cup of broth to loosen the vegetables and prevent sticking.

Add the turkey and cook, separating into bite-size pieces with a wooden spatula, for about 5 to 7 minutes, until the meat is cooked all the way through (don't overcook). Add 1 teaspoon salt and the Bragg Liquid Aminos, dill, thyme, and asafetida and stir until the mixture is uniform.

Add $2/3$ cup of broth and bring to a boil. Reduce the heat to low and add the flour. Stir for about 1 minute, until the mixture thickens. Remove from the heat and cover the pan.

When the potatoes are cooked, drain and mash with butter, or oil if you want to make your cottage pie dairy-free. Add salt to taste. Whip the potatoes using a handheld mixer and adding the remaining ⅓ cup hot broth gradually, until the mashed potatoes reach the desired fluffiness.

Serve immediately in a bowl with the turkey mixture on the bottom and mashed potatoes on top. Garnish with dill.

Note: The cottage pie can be reserved overnight. To reheat, preheat the oven to 400°F. Layer the turkey mixture and potatoes in a small casserole dish, cover with foil, and bake for 10 to 15 minutes, until the pie is piping hot, and serve.

FRESH FISH EN PAPILLOTE WITH POTATOES, OLIVES, AND LEEKS (AP)

Serves 2   Prep and cooking time: 30 minutes

In French, *en papillote* refers to baking food in a pouch made of parchment paper, though in a pinch a heavy-duty foil cinched at the top will do just as well. Perfect for a weeknight dinner, this rustic dish is a wholesome and easy way to bring together fish and potatoes with a few aromatics for a warm and satisfying meal. A mild-flavored, thick-fleshed fish such as cod or mullet works well for this recipe. For a special meal, a fillet of skinned branzino, a Mediterranean fish that is slightly more expensive but very delicate and flavorful, will produce wonders. For Acid Watchers craving the tartness of citrus, this dish allows you to use fresh lemon juice—but only if it is applied to uncooked fish as part of a marinade. Raw animal protein can absorb the pepsin-activating acidity of the lemon but will allow it to retain the tang of freshness that goes so well with all seafood. I like to use fingerling or multicolored small potatoes in the papillote because they have less starch and more flavor than more common varieties. But don't make a special run to the store if you don't have any on hand; a quartered Yukon Gold potato will work well enough. Leave the potato skin on for extra fiber.

> 10 fingerling potatoes or 2 small, quartered Yukon Gold
>   potatoes, washed
> ½ teaspoon Celtic salt, plus more to taste

2 (6-ounce) fillets of cod, mullet, or branzino

Juice of 1 lemon

1 teaspoon olive oil

2 ounces leeks (approximately 1 cup; white part only), thoroughly washed and cut into rings

1 tablespoon chopped fresh parsley

1 teaspoon organic butter

Whole fresh parsley leaves, for garnish

$^1/_4$ teaspoon ground sumac

2 tablespoons pitted niçoise olives, drained and chopped

Preheat the oven to 400°F. Place a parchment or foil pouch on a baking sheet.

Bring the potatoes to a boil in a small pot of generously salted water. Reduce the heat to low and simmer for 10 minutes. Drain and dry the potatoes.

While the potatoes are cooking, dry the fish fillets with a paper towel, season them with $^1/_2$ teaspoon salt on both sides, and drizzle with the lemon juice and oil.

In the parchment or foil pouch, layer the potatoes, fish fillets, leeks, chopped parsley, and butter. Bake for 10 to 12 minutes, until the fish has released its juices and becomes flaky.

Remove the baking sheet from the oven and open the pouch. Be careful not to burn your hands on the steam coming from the contents of the pouch.

Allow the pouch to rest for 3 to 5 minutes. Carefully transfer the pouch onto a serving dish, taking care not to spill the juices. Sprinkle with the whole parsley leaves, sumac, and olives. Serve immediately.

MAINTENANCE PHASE SIDE DISHES

SAUTÉ OF FENNEL, RED CABBAGE, AND SWISS CHARD (V)

Serves 4 to 6   Prep and cooking time: 35 to 45 minutes

This easy-to-prepare but abundant-in-taste side dish complements any protein serving and serves particularly well as a base for grilled fish or flank steak. It contains a minimal number of ingredients and is simple to make. The trick to making it extra delicious is to sauté the vegetables one at a time, as each requires different cooking time for optimal results. Another tip: don't toss the Swiss chard stalks, especially if you are using the red variety. They add a beautiful spark of red to the dish of green, purple, and white.

> 3 tablespoons coconut oil
> 2 fennel bulbs, cored, outer layer removed, halved and thinly sliced, fronds reserved
> $1/2$ medium head red cabbage, outer leaves removed, cored, and thinly sliced
> Celtic salt, to taste
> Bunch of Swiss chard, washed thoroughly and chopped, stalks reserved and finely chopped
> $1/4$ teaspoon caraway seeds
> $1/2$ teaspoon ground sumac

In a nonstick pan, heat 1 tablespoon of the oil over medium heat. Stir-fry the sliced fennel for 5 to 7 minutes, until the slices begin to caramelize. Remove from the pan.

Add 1 tablespoon of the oil to the same pan, raise the heat to high, and sauté the cabbage for 2 minutes. Sprinkle with salt and add $1/4$ cup water. Reduce the heat to medium, cover the pan, and allow the cabbage to steam for 8 minutes.

Add the Swiss chard and caraway seeds to the cabbage. Stir, cover the pan, and sauté for 3 to 5 minutes more. Remove from the heat.

Return the fennel into the pan. Sprinkle with the reserved fennel fronds and sumac and serve.

KALE "COBB" SALAD (V)
Serves 4 to 6   Prep and cooking time: 1 hour

A traditional Cobb salad is an assembled salad that is built on a base of lettuce and tomatoes and taken up several notches with avocado, chicken or seafood, blue cheese, a sprinkling of bacon, and hard-boiled eggs, and then smothered in rich, vinegar-infused dressing. Unfortunately, it is not an Acid Watcher's friend. My Kale "Cobb" Salad uses the salad's distinct range of textures—creamy and crunchy—to make a filling meal. A serving of grilled chicken, shrimp, salmon, or lobster makes it complete. Or enjoy it vegan style.

$^1/_3$ cup dry French green lentils

1 dried bay leaf

Celtic salt, to taste

$^1/_3$ cup spelt berries, soaked in water for 30 minutes

12 to 15 green beans

1 bunch Tuscan kale, washed thoroughly, stems removed

2 ounces finely chopped feta cheese

1 tablespoon toasted sunflower seeds

$^1/_2$ Hass avocado, pitted, scooped, and diced

1 tablespoon olive oil

$^1/_2$ teaspoon ground sumac

In a medium pot, bring the lentils to a boil with 1 cup water, the bay leaf, and salt. Reduce the heat to low, cover, and simmer for 22 to 25 minutes, until all the water is absorbed. Discard the bay leaf.

Rinse the soaked spelt berries and bring them to a boil in a separate pot with $1^1/_2$ cups salted water. Reduce the heat and simmer for 22 to 24 minutes, until all the water is absorbed and the spelt berries are chewy.

While the lentils and spelt berries are simmering, blanch the green beans. (See page 135 for blanching instructions.) Chop finely.

In the same pot, blanch the kale. Kale is very watery, so after draining, remove all of the remaining water from the kale by squeezing the leaves out by hand. Finely chop the kale.

In a large bowl, combine the lentils, spelt berries, green beans, kale, feta cheese, sunflower seeds, and avocado and toss with the oil, sumac, and more salt, if needed. Serve immediately.

BRUSSELS SPROUT SALAD WITH PECANS, RAISINS, AND APPLE (V)

Serves 2   Prep and cooking time: 25 minutes

In the past, Brussels sprouts have gotten a bum rap, mostly from people who had the misfortune of tasting them steamed or poached to bitter limpness. Brussels sprouts are at their tastiest when raw and shredded, or when they are roasted, a cooking process that takes the bitterness out and adds smokiness and crunch to balance their chewy texture. When in season and roasted, Brussels sprouts are a delicious accompaniment to any comfort meal. As an ingredient in this salad, this elegant vegetable neutralizes the acidity of the apple. Raisins add a burst of sweetness and pecans a dose of omega fats to keep bad food cravings away.

> 1 pound Brussels sprouts, trimmed and sliced
> Celtic salt, to taste
> 1 apple, cored and thinly sliced or chopped into $1/2$-inch pieces
> $1/2$ cup chopped raw pecans
> $1/2$ cup raisins
> 2 teaspoons olive oil

Preheat the oven to 350°F. Spread the Brussels sprouts on a baking sheet and sprinkle with salt. Roast for 10 to 15 minutes, until they are still crunchy but slightly toasted on the outside.

Toss the Brussels sprouts with the apple, pecans, raisins, oil, and salt, and serve.

MAINTENANCE PHASE STOCKS

HOMEMADE CHICKEN BROTH (AP)
Makes 12 cups (24 servings)
Prep and cooking time: 30 minutes, plus 2 hours for
simmering and more for cooling

You may have heard chicken soup referred to as "Jewish penicillin," and if you've ever sipped its clear broth while sick, you have probably experienced the time-tested curative magic for which it is renowned. Homemade chicken broth is an excellent, low-calorie, high-nutrient source of protein, vitamins, and minerals. It can be enjoyed on its own or serve as a base for an endless variety of soups. Reduced to a stock, it can accent stews, sauces, and braised dishes. While a deliciously rich chicken broth takes a long time to simmer to perfection, the prep work is quick and easy to master. Because broth can be made in big batches and stored in a freezer, it is a low-budget, long-lasting meal helper.

For optimal health benefits and flavor, use organic or kosher chicken—while it is more expensive, keep in mind that the broth will yield at least 12 servings. By choosing organic you'll do your Acid Watcher duty of eliminating the additives, hormones, and antibiotics that contribute to oxidative stress. There is, however, a way to have the "organic" experience without the cost by opting for chicken backs, necks, and feet instead of the whole chicken. Not only is "bone broth"—which is being rediscovered by a new generation of foodies—less expensive, it actually produces a thicker, tastier broth thanks to all the collagen in the bones. Some high-end grocery chains like Whole Foods offer bones as a selection among other poultry offerings. But if you don't see the bones for sale, you can always ask the butcher to give you some. They are always sold at a discount.

1 (3- to 4-pound) kosher or organic whole chicken, cut into
    8 pieces, breast meat removed and reserved for other use, or
    3 to 4 pounds chicken backs, necks, and feet
About 3 quarts filtered water
1 large yellow onion

2 leeks (white parts only), thoroughly washed

1 fennel bulb, stems, fronds, and outer shell

1 carrot

2 celery stalks

1 small turnip, peeled

1 small parsnip, peeled

Asparagus ends (optional)

$1/2$ cup fresh parsley and dill leaves and/or stems

1 tablespoon Celtic salt, more if needed

Wash the chicken and trim the fat off, or wash the backs, necks, and feet, if using.

Spread the chicken parts along the bottom of a 5-quart pot and pour in the filtered water. The chicken should be fully submerged with an inch or two to spare. Bring to a rapid boil.

While the water comes to a boil, roughly chop the onion, leeks, fennel, carrot, celery, turnip, parsnip, and asparagus ends.

Reduce to a simmer and skim the residue that comes up to the surface using a slotted spoon. When the broth is as clear as you can make it, add the vegetables, parsley, and dill, raise the heat to high, and bring to a second boil.

Reduce to a simmer and skim any additional fat.

Add salt, cover the pot, and simmer for 2 hours, checking on the broth two or three times and removing any residue that continues to come up. (Kosher and organic chicken will produce less fat and residue than their counterparts.)

Remove from the heat and allow the broth to cool to room temperature. Add salt to taste.

Strain the broth through a fine-mesh sieve. Reserve the meat from the whole chicken (if using) for Pesto Chicken Sandwich (page 167), Colorful Chicken Salad (page 170), or to enjoy by itself. Discard the bones and vegetables.

VEGETABLE STOCK (V)
Makes 2 quarts
Prep and cooking time: 1 hour 40 minutes, plus more for soaking mushrooms and cooling

This versatile broth flavors rice, quinoa, buckwheat groats, and other soups. Divide into batches and store in the freezer for up to 1 month.

$2^1/_2$ ounces dried wild mushrooms (porcini, shiitake, or a combination)

Stems of fresh shiitake mushrooms (optional)

2 medium onions

1 medium leek (white part only), thoroughly washed

1 medium parsnip, peeled and roughly chopped

1 fennel bulb, stalks, fronds, and outer shell

1 bunch cilantro, stems only, washed and trimmed

2 carrots, roughly chopped

2 celery stalks, chopped

$^1/_3$ medium turnip, peeled and roughly chopped

$^1/_4$ medium rutabaga, peeled and roughly chopped

3 quarts filtered water

2 teaspoons Celtic salt

Soak the dried mushrooms in a bowl filled with water for at least 4 hours or overnight.

Drain the mushrooms, reserving 2 cups soaking liquid.

Combine the soaked mushrooms and the shiitake stems, onions, leek, parsnip, fennel, cilantro stems, carrots, celery, turnip, and rutabaga in a 5-quart pot. Fill with the filtered water and add the salt.

Bring to a high boil. Reduce the heat, cover, and simmer for 1 hour.

Remove from the heat and allow to cool completely.

Drain the broth into a large bowl and discard the vegetables.

MAINTENANCE PHASE DESSERTS

ACID WATCHER CHUNKY MONKEY COOKIES (E)
Makes 10 to 15 cookies
Prep and cooking time: 45 minutes, plus 4 hours for cooling

This variation on the traditional chocolate chip cookie will be familiar in taste but original in presentation. Carob chips don't hold up to oven heat as well as chocolate chips, so the best way to use them is as a ganache filling placed between two thin cookies, with a macadamia nut on top. It makes for a rich, crunchy, and creamy bite of a dessert that you won't believe is Acid Watcher–friendly and low in sugar when you taste it. Be careful when rolling out the dough. Healthier whole-wheat flour makes for a slightly more delicate batter, but it more than stands up in taste. And don't overdo the filling; carob ganache can be runnier than chocolate, especially at room temperature.

$1/2$ cup carob chips

$1/3$ cup almond milk

4 ounces organic butter (1 stick), at room temperature

$1/3$ cup organic agave nectar

1 large egg

$1/2$ teaspoon vanilla extract

$1^1/3$ cups whole-wheat flour, plus more for dusting

Dash of Celtic salt

$1/4$ teaspoon baking soda

15 macadamia nuts

Melt the carob chips with the almond milk in a double boiler (or a glass bowl positioned over a pan with boiling water) by whisking the mixture until it is smooth and syrupy. Cool and refrigerate the ganache for at least 4 hours, or overnight.

Preheat the oven to 375°F.

Line a large baking sheet with parchment paper.

Using a handheld mixer, whip the butter and agave nectar on medium speed for 2 minutes. Add the egg and vanilla and mix on low speed for another minute, until the mixture is uniform.

In a separate bowl, whisk the flour, salt, and baking soda.

Using a handheld mixer, combine the wet and dry ingredients and mix on low speed for 1 to 2 minutes, until the dough is thick and gooey. Using your hands, shape the dough into a ball, cover, and refrigerate for 30 minutes.

On a large board, use a rolling pin dusted with flour to carefully roll out the dough to about 1/2 inch thick.

Cut out about 30 cookies using a water glass or a cookie cutter. Mount a macadamia nut in the center of half of the cookies (see note), planting it firmly into the dough.

Bake for 10 minutes. Allow to cool completely.

Using a teaspoon, place a small amount of carob ganache on a flat surface of each cookie without a nut, and make a "sandwich" by placing a cookie with a nut on top.

Repeat until all the cookies are assembled. Refrigerate before serving.

Note: Depending on the size of the cookie cutter, you may end up with fewer than 30 cookies. That's okay; the important part is that you have an even number of cookies.

GREEK YOGURT PARFAIT WITH DRIED CHERRY COMPOTE, HONEY, AND ALMONDS (D)
Serves 4   Prep and cooking time: 25 minutes

In the United States we are accustomed to eating fruit and yogurt for breakfast, but in some Mediterranean cultures you are more likely to see it served as a light dessert. To satisfy a sweet tooth, you are much better off enjoying it at the end of a nice meal rather than at the beginning of the day. This fruit-and-yogurt dish is optimal in flavor and health benefits unlike what you can buy at the grocery store, after it has been preserved, processed, and acidified. It is also much prettier, and it is very easy to make. If you don't have almonds on hand, macadamia nuts and walnuts are a great alternative. (You don't have to toast macadamia nuts to get the full flavor.)

> 4 ounces dried cherries
> 1 cup filtered water
> 1/2 teaspoon arrowroot powder
> 2 cups plain Greek yogurt (Greek Gods or Fage 2% brand)
> 1/2 cup toasted blanched and slivered almonds (see note)
> 1 to 2 tablespoons honey for drizzling

In a small pot, bring the cherries and filtered water to a boil. Reduce the heat to low and simmer for 15 minutes. Remove from the heat.

In a separate bowl, make a slurry of 1 tablespoon of the cherry cooking liquid and the arrowroot powder. Whisk until smooth.

Pour the slurry back into the pot with the cherries, stir, and bring to room temperature. The mixture will thicken gradually.

To serve, place a dollop of yogurt at the bottom of each bowl. Add a layer of cherries. Add another layer of yogurt on top. Sprinkle with toasted almonds and drizzle with honey.

Note: To toast almonds, preheat a small pan over medium-low heat. Toast the almonds for 5 minutes, until they start browning and releasing their aroma. Be careful not to burn the almonds.

APPLE CROSTATA (F)
Serves 8 to 10
Prep time: 40 minutes, plus more for baking and cooling

This rustic, simpler-than-it-sounds dessert is an Acid Watcher alternative to the more traditional apple pies and tarts. A touch of cardamom and goat cheese gives it uniqueness and depth.

PASTRY SHELL
> 8 tablespoons (1 stick) unsalted organic butter, plus more for greasing the pan, at room temperature

1^{1}/3 cups whole-wheat flour, plus more for dusting

^{1}/2 cup almond flour

^{1}/4 cup agave nectar

^{1}/2 cup almond milk

^{1}/2 teaspoon vanilla extract

Celtic salt, to taste

FILLING

1 tablespoon almond flour

1 tablespoon whole-wheat flour

1 tablespoon agave nectar

^{1}/3 cup walnuts

2 tablespoons organic unsalted butter

^{1}/4 teaspoon ground cardamom

4 ounces goat cheese

1 large egg, at room temperature

2 Golden Delicious apples

^{1}/2 teaspoon ground cinnamon

Preheat the oven to 375°F. Grease and flour a round baking sheet, preferably a 9-inch pizza dish.

Make the pastry: Using a pastry blender, combine the butter, whole-wheat flour, almond flour, and agave nectar until the mixture is coarse. Add the almond milk, vanilla, and salt, and blend.

Mold the dough into a ball with your hands, adding more whole-wheat flour if necessary to prevent it from sticking. Put the dough back into the bowl, cover with plastic wrap, and refrigerate for 30 minutes.

Make the filling: While the dough is chilling, combine the filling ingredients in a food processor and pulse until the mixture is creamy and uniform. Place in a bowl, cover with plastic wrap, and refrigerate until you are ready to complete the crostata.

Dust a large cutting board and a rolling pin with whole-wheat flour. Remove the dough from the refrigerator and carefully roll it out into a circle (it doesn't have to be precise) slightly larger than the baking sheet.

The dough will be flaky. Carefully transfer the dough onto the baking sheet.

Prepare the apples by halving them, coring them, and slicing them into thin strips. You have to move quickly as the apples will soon oxidize.

Remove the filling from the refrigerator. Using a flat, thin spatula, spread the filling on top of the dough. Place the apple slices in concentric circles and crimp the overhanging dough to create a rim around the crostata.

Place into the oven on the center rack and bake for 45 to 50 minutes, until the apples are crisp around the edges and the filling is bubbly.

Remove from the oven and cool completely. Sprinkle with cinnamon and serve.

LUXURIOUS "CHOCOLATE" TORTE (D)
Serves 6 to 8
Prep and cooking time: 20 minutes for the cake,
7 minutes for the frosting, plus baking and cooling time

This decadent torte would not be considered appropriate for calorie-reduction diets, but it is consistent with the Acid Watcher principles of no white flour, no processed sugar, no milk, and no chocolate. Yet it looks and tastes like the chocolate cake of your dreams. Because the cake doesn't have wheat flour, it is fragile, so be careful when transporting.

CAKE

8 tablespoons (1 stick) organic unsalted butter, plus more for greasing the pan, at room temperature

1/4 cup agave nectar

2 large eggs, at room temperature

1 teaspoon vanilla extract

1/3 cup full-fat plain Greek yogurt

1/4 cup almond milk

1 cup almond flour, plus more for dusting

$^1/_3$ cup coconut flour

$^1/_4$ cup carob powder

$^1/_2$ teaspoon baking soda

1 teaspoon baking powder

Dash of Celtic salt

FROSTING

$^1/_2$ cup almond milk

1 cup carob chips

$^1/_4$ teaspoon vanilla extract

$^1/_4$ teaspoon ground cinnamon

$^1/_2$ teaspoon carob powder

Dash of Celtic salt

8 tablespoons (1 stick) organic unsalted butter, at room
temperature

Preheat the oven to 350°F. Grease and flour a parchment-lined, 8-inch springform pan.

Make the cake: In a large glass bowl, use a handheld mixer to whip the butter and agave nectar for 2 minutes. Add the eggs, one at a time, and continue mixing. Don't overmix. Whisk in the vanilla, yogurt, and almond milk.

In a separate bowl, sift the almond flour, coconut flour, carob powder, baking soda, baking powder, and salt. Combine the wet and dry ingredients by folding the dry ingredients into the wet ingredients a third at a time.

Pour the batter—which will be thick—into the springform pan, evening it out as much as possible.

Bake for 25 to 30 minutes, until the middle of the cake is cooked through. (Test by inserting a toothpick into the center. The toothpick should be dry when it comes out.)

Make the frosting: Bring water to a boil in a double boiler and reduce to a simmer. Place the almond milk, carob chips, vanilla, cinnamon, carob powder, and salt in the top of the double boiler and allow to melt, whisking to prevent burning. This should take 3 to 5 minutes. Remove from the heat immediately and place in a glass bowl. Cool to room temperature.

When the frosting has cooled to room temperature, add the butter. Using a handheld mixer, mix on high speed until the frosting is consistent and smooth.

When the cake has cooled but is still warm, about 20 minutes, release the sides of the pan. Spread half of the frosting on the cake while it is warm so it can absorb the rich flavor. Refrigerate the rest of the frosting for 1 to 2 hours. Complete the frosting process when the cake has cooled completely and the frosting has completed chilling.

Serve immediately. Refrigerate leftovers, if any.

FRUIT KABOBS WITH CAROB FONDUE (F)
Serves 2
Prep and cooking time: 5 to 7 minutes, plus more for cleaning and/or chopping fruit

This is one of the more low-maintenance dessert options for the Maintenance Phase. Whole strawberries, pineapple chunks, and banana slices make the best presentation. Serve the fruit on a platter with a bowl of fondue on the side. Thread fruit pieces on a wooden skewer or serve with small picks inserted into individual fruit pieces. Dip into the fondue, and enjoy!

$1/3$ cup carob chips

1 tablespoon carob powder

$1/3$ cup almond milk

Bring water to a gentle boil in a double boiler. Reduce the heat to medium-high.

Combine all of the ingredients in the top of the double boiler and simmer, whisking vigorously, for 2 to 4 minutes, until the mixture melts and turns smooth. Remove from the heat and transfer to a serving bowl.

AFTER-DINNER CHEESE PLATE (D)

For Acid Watchers who have a taste for dessert but prefer the less sugary variety, an after-dinner cheese plate is an elegant option. (That's how they still eat dessert in the Mediterranean region!) What makes a dessert cheese plate different from the more familiar hors d'oeuvre presentation is the accent on fresh and dried fruit, nuts, and sweeteners that are served with the cheeses. To make your cheese plate complex and colorful, serve three varieties of Acid Watcher–approved cheeses—for example, Asiago, Cheddar, and blue cheese—accompanied by dried apricots or cherries for dried fruit; apples, pears, or grapes for fresh fruit; pecans and blanched hazelnuts or almonds for nuts. Include a small honey pot for drizzling (softer cheeses and honey go well together) and whole-grain toasts for serving.

COCONUT-CARROT BARS (D)

Serves 12   Prep and cooking time: 50 minutes

This low-sugar, low-acid variation on an American classic dessert can be enjoyed naked (that is, without the frosting!) or, for a special occasion, with a frosting of whipped mascarpone, a more delicate, less-processed Italian version of cream cheese.

BARS

- 8 tablespoons (1 stick) organic unsalted butter, at room temperature, plus more for greasing the pan
- 1 cup almond flour, plus more for dusting
- $1/2$ cup coconut flour
- 1 teaspoon baking powder
- 1 teaspoon baking soda
- $1^1/2$ teaspoons ground cinnamon, plus more for frosting (optional)
- $1/4$ teaspoon ground allspice
- $1/4$ teaspoon ground cloves

Dash of Celtic salt

1/4 cup agave nectar

4 large eggs

1 teaspoon vanilla extract

3 medium carrots, finely grated

2 inches fresh ginger, peeled and grated

FROSTING (OPTIONAL)

8 ounce container mascarpone cream

2 tablespoons coconut milk

2 tablespoons agave nectar

1/2 teaspoon vanilla extract

Preheat the oven to 350°F. Prepare a 9 by 9-inch baking dish by greasing it with butter and dusting it with almond flour.

Make the bars: Sift the almond flour, coconut flour, baking powder, baking soda, cinnamon, allspice, cloves, and salt into a large bowl.

In a separate bowl, use a handheld mixer to whip the butter and agave nectar on medium speed for 2 minutes. Add the eggs, one at a time. The mixture will look a little lumpy, but don't overmix. Stir in the vanilla.

Combine the wet and dry ingredients and fold in the carrots and ginger. Carefully pour the batter into the baking dish. Use a spatula to even out the mixture. The layer will be thin.

Bake for 30 minutes, remove from the oven, and allow to cool completely.

Make the frosting (if using): In a small bowl, use a handheld mixer to whip the mascarpone on high speed until fluffy.

Add the coconut milk, a tablespoon at a time, to thin the frosting. Whisk in the agave nectar and vanilla until the mixture is smooth. Refrigerate if not using immediately.

Frost with mascarpone cream, if using, and sprinkle with cinnamon. Divide into 16 bars and serve immediately (see note).

Note: If the bars are frosted, keep refrigerated until ready to serve.

ZUCCHINI MUFFINS WITH "CHOCOLATE" GANACHE (G)

Serves 12

Prep and cooking time: 20 minutes, plus more for cooling

Peculiar as it sounds, zucchini and chocolate is a Mediterranean-style marriage made in culinary heaven, but in this Acid Watcher version, zucchini is paired with carob ganache. You won't taste zucchini in your muffin, but it will make it delectably moist. Naturally sweetened with agave nectar and dairy free, this is a go-to treat for any time of day.

$2/3$ cup coconut oil, melted over low heat and cooled to room temperature

$1/3$ cup agave nectar

2 large eggs

1 teaspoon vanilla extract

$1^1/2$ cups whole-wheat flour

$1/2$ teaspoon baking soda

$1/2$ teaspoon baking powder

Pinch of Celtic salt

$1/2$ teaspoon ground cinnamon

$1/2$ cup walnuts, pulsed in a food processor to flour consistency

1 zucchini, washed thoroughly, ends trimmed, finely grated

Preheat the oven to 350°F. Set up paper liners in a 12-cup muffin pan.

In a medium bowl, whisk the oil, agave nectar, eggs, and vanilla.

Sift the flour, baking soda, baking powder, salt, and cinnamon into a small bowl.

Combine the wet and dry ingredients. Fold in the walnuts and zucchini.

Divide the batter among the cupcake liners, filling them approximately halfway to the top.

Bake for 20 minutes. Cool completely.

Frost, if desired, with carob ganache (page 191) and serve immediately.

CHAPTER 12

Getting pHit

WHAT YOU NEED TO KNOW ABOUT EXERCISE
FOR ACID REFLUX DISEASE

Given the digestive origins of acid damage, it would be easy to overlook exercise as part of the solution to your reflux-related symptoms. But it shouldn't be discounted. Although eating a low-acid, high-fiber diet will be the most powerful tool for reversing acid damage and alleviating reflux symptoms, exercise can help produce profound improvements beyond those that you might experience by following the diet alone.

When it comes to your health, the importance of creating (or maintaining) a consistent exercise habit cannot be overstated. Exercise has many benefits, such as helping your cells use glucose more efficiently, thereby balancing blood sugar, and reducing blood vessel stiffness, which can lower blood pressure by letting blood flow more freely. Exercise can also help lower levels of triglycerides and LDL cholesterol, both of which have been linked to a greater risk for developing heart disease. Unlike medications that promise these same benefits, exercise doesn't come with any baggage (unless you count your gym bag). There are typically no negative side effects associated with breaking a sweat, with the caveat being that you should consult with your doctor before undertaking any type of exercise regimen.

As an Acid Watcher, you should note that the risk of esophageal cancer has been shown to be 29 percent lower in those who are most physically active when compared to those who are least active. This could be related to the fact that exercise can help you reach and maintain a healthy weight, which could ward off continued or future acid damage, including the type that can set the stage for cancer of the esophagus. Exercise will also benefit you by helping to neutralize stress hormones such as cortisol, which we know can turn up the production of both gastric acid and pepsin.

Increased physical activity can improve sleep quality and duration. Lack of sleep has been significantly associated with acid reflux disease, and the reverse is certainly true, too—many people with acid reflux and throatburn reflux regularly lose sleep because of the discomfort or disruption caused by their symptoms. You will alleviate some symptoms of nighttime reflux if you follow the rule of letting three hours go between your last meal of the day and bedtime, but a specific exercise approach can also subdue postmeal acid activity.

Importantly, a consistent exercise habit will help accelerate weight loss, which can lessen the type of gastric pressure that leaves you vulnerable to refluxed acid. It can also rejuvenate you in an unexpected way, and help further energize your efforts to eat best for your health.

I personally experienced these exercise perks after finally being turned on to fitness in 2007 (it's amazing what seeing a photo of yourself with a Buddha belly can do). My dedication then to a calisthenics-based boot camp helped me lose forty-eight pounds and drop six inches from my waist. My work in the gym motivated me to work just as hard on my diet, which centered on some of the key dietary principles featured in the Acid Watcher Diet: no alcohol, especially in the early stages, and no processed foods full of sugar and preservatives. The combined efforts helped me recapture an energy that I thought had faded alongside my younger years into the past.

The good news is that you don't have to do a strenuous boot camp to experience the benefits of exercise. In fact, during the Healing Phase, you may want to consider curtailing any extended sessions of vigorous exercise, as prolonged exertion can aggravate and even trigger acid reflux symptoms. For our purposes, the intensity of the exercise is not as crucial as the regularity with which you pursue it. There are other special precautions and considerations for exercising with acid reflux.

The Dos and Don'ts of Exercising with Acid Reflux Disease

DO MAKE YOUR EXERCISE HABIT CONSISTENT

Compared to an inconsistent habit, regular exercise is more likely to help promote weight loss (or weight maintenance if you're already at a healthy weight) and lower your BMI. This is because exercise will help burn at least some of the calories you consume each day by using them as fuel rather than letting them go unused. When calories go unused, they don't just sit idle like a pile of clean laundry waiting to be folded when you have time—they get stored in your fat cells for later use and you gain weight. The longer this calories-stored-as-fat cycle continues, the more difficult, thanks to age-related slowing of metabolism, it becomes to burn off accumulated fat tissue. This is why it's better to exercise off unused calories today than to find them around your waist tomorrow.

You can lose weight through diet alone, but research tells us that combining diet and exercise creates more sustained weight loss, and a review of over 490 studies on diet and exercise revealed that people who combined efforts maintained weight loss better than those who only introduced dietary changes. Exercise can help change your body composition in ways that diet alone can't, especially by adding muscle, which burns more calories than any other type of tissue.

How much exercise do you need? The minimum recommended amount is 150 minutes a week of physical activity, which is approximately 21 minutes a day or a little over 40 minutes every other day. Because exercise has a cumulative effect on metabolism, motivation, and endurance, it's recommended that you don't go more than one day without getting in some type of workout. In other words, don't try to save up your 150 minutes for one weekend day—spread it out throughout the week. While there are immediate gains from exercise, they tend not to last more than a day or so. The goal is to never stray too far from the endorphins and other mood-boosting brain chemicals that can improve your overall well-being and remind you just how invigorating exercise can be.

If you feel too tired to dedicate time to exercise, consider this: once you start exercising, you'll find that you have more energy. I'm speaking from both clinical research and personal experience. Exhaustion is caused in large part by the draining duo of too much stress and too little sleep, one usually leading to the other and then back again. Exercise has proven to help people with anxiety fall asleep faster and stay asleep for longer periods of time. It has also shown to be an effective drug-free way to treat sleep disorders in people age sixty and older. Make time for exercise in your life and you'll soon be getting better sleep, enjoying more energy, and feeling more motivated than ever to stay on track with your dietary commitments.

DO LEARN TO LOVE POST-MEAL WALKS

When you eat and drink, your stomach naturally expands to make room for what you've just ingested, which can increase pressure on the lower esophageal sphincter (LES) and lead to a relaxing of this important muscle. As you know by now, once this muscle relaxes, the doorway to refluxed acid has been precariously left open. One way to prevent the gastric distention that occurs after you eat from placing too much pressure on the LES is to simply go for a walk after meals. This can minimize the pressure by helping accelerate digestive processes, which will empty the stomach and shrink it back to size at a faster rate. It's likely because of this effect on digestion that a post-dinner walk has been linked to reduced risk of stomach cancer.

As an Acid Watcher, you should make a stroll after supper a priority as often as possible, because it will be good for both your reflux and your mind (walking is a bona fide stress soother). If you have a dog that gets walked once or twice a day, consider making one of those outings happen after dinner. You can certainly walk after other meals as well if you'd like, but the timing of the nighttime walk is important, as it should also lessen your chances of experiencing nocturnal reflux. To help ensure that this walk prevents rather than provokes refluxed acid, it's best to stick to a leisurely pace, which should be decidedly slower than the brisk or vigorous one you will aim for during exercise.

DO PRACTICE DIAPHRAGMATIC BREATHING

There is growing evidence that diaphragmatic breathing exercises can help strengthen the tendons of the diaphragm that overlap near the lower esophageal sphincter, leading to an increase in the overall pressure around the esophageal junction and creating a stronger barrier against refluxed acid. Diaphragmatic breathing is also known as abdominal breathing because the focus during this type of respiration is your belly instead of your chest (if you inhale and exhale right now you'll notice that most of the movement takes place in your chest).

A study published in the *American Journal of Gastroenterology* revealed that abdominal breathing had a positive effect on reflux symptoms and reduced the need for reflux medication in people with GERD. The results were promising, but the researchers also discovered that nearly half of the people participating in the study had a tough time sticking with the exercises, which required a thirty-minute commitment each day. For this reason, I'm sharing with you here some basic instructions on how to practice diaphragmatic breathing, but with no specific or strict protocol. I encourage you to try it even for just five to ten breaths each day and see if it produces any benefits for you. If nothing else, a few moments dedicated to deep breathing exercises might diminish feelings of stress and leave you with a renewed sense of calm.

To practice diaphragmatic breathing, first get into a comfortable starting position. This could be lying down on your back with your knees bent and feet on the floor, sitting on a chair that allows your feet to be flat on the ground, or standing with your feet hip-width apart. In either position, focus on keeping your spine erect as you place one hand on your chest and one hand just at your beltline. Inhale deeply and slowly through your nose, taking air into your belly (you'll know you're doing it right if the hand at your beltline rises). Exhale through your nose, feeling your belly as it sinks back in. Repeat five to ten times, alternating the position of your hands if you'd like. Belly breathing can be practiced at any time of day and can serve as a nice breath of fresh air during your lunch or coffee break.

DO TRY A GENTLE YOGA CLASS

If you've never tried it, yoga may seem intimidating. And for good reason—it can appear as though you need to be some type of contortionist to even get in the room. In truth, yoga is for anybody who's interested in gaining flexibility, strength, and balance. If you are a beginner, try hatha yoga, which is a broad category of practice that focuses on learning yoga poses that promote stability, strength, and controlled breathing. Of these, the Iyengar style emphasizes proper alignment, which is crucial to master if you want to progress to more advanced practice, including the popular Vinyasa or Bikram variations, to name a few. Low-impact yoga practice can be good for people with acid reflux because its emphasis on deep breathing, flexibility, and mindfulness can help cool down stress hormones that increase acid production.

Look for a gentle or beginner yoga class, preferably at a smaller studio rather than a gym. Studio classes typically have a smaller class size, increasing your chances of getting personal instruction, and are usually taught by instructors whose primary focus is yoga rather than other types of exercise. You'll want an instructor who will make sure that your poses are done correctly for maximal benefit. As a person with acid reflux, you must avoid certain poses, such as inversions. These include headstands or handstands (which you are unlikely to encounter in a beginner class). You should also pay attention to the most ubiquitous pose, the downward dog, to see if you notice any reflux symptoms. For some, this position, which requires the head to be positioned below the waist, will trigger symptoms. Others will be fine. Pay attention to your personal response to different poses and ask the instructor for modifications as needed. Good instructors will always ask new students if they have any physical conditions that the instructor should be aware of before the start of practice. If you experience chronic heartburn, make sure your instructor is aware.

DO MEASURE YOUR "WAIST LOSS" IF YOU WANT TO TRACK YOUR PROGRESS

When you combine regular exercise with the dietary principles of the Acid Watcher Diet, you will lose total body weight, including weight from your abdominal region. Weight loss from your middle, especially that which comes from the deeper visceral fat, is an important marker of positive internal changes that are taking place. Research reveals that this type of belly fat may not be as stubborn as you think: as little as 5 to 10 percent of initial total weight loss has shown to reduce visceral fat by 10 to 30 percent. Reducing visceral fat can do the following:

- Reduce levels of inflammatory markers that are produced by this type of metabolically active belly fat
- Improve factors related to metabolic syndrome, which exacerbate inflammation
- Reduce risk for Barrett esophagus; a strong association between the precancerous condition and central obesity has been noted in several studies

You can measure your waist loss in whichever way you'd prefer. A tape measure will provide a precise marker by which to measure progress. Using this method, simply run the tape measure around your waist at belly button level and note the number of inches. You can also use an item of clothing, such as a pair of jeans, to gauge weight lost from your waist. This is a decidedly less scientific method, but it's simple and allows you to truly feel your progress. Another option is to use your belt, if you wear one regularly. Make note of your starting notch and then monitor your progress by notch changes that occur as you make your way through the program. Of course, if you find that you're loosening your belt rather than tightening it, you may want to take stock of your processed food intake.

DON'T EXERCISE UNTIL IT'S BEEN TWO TO THREE HOURS SINCE YOU'VE EATEN

In chapter 8, you learned that gravity can be a formidable foe against comfort in postmeal reclining, especially if the digestion process in the stomach hasn't been completed. The same logic applies to exercise. If you try to exercise on a full or even partly full stomach, there is a greater risk that certain movements or types of movement will lead to increased pressure on the LES, which if compromised will let in gastric acid and tissue-damaging pepsin. To prevent this from happening, be sure to exercise only after at least two hours have passed since you've eaten, and three hours for larger meals. Depending on your schedule, this may require you to work out on an empty stomach before breakfast. If you are completing activities at moderate intensity, this should be fine, but as always pay attention to how you feel. Try to drink 16 ounces of water (about two glasses) upon rising to ensure that your body is hydrated before you start exercising. Avoid drinking coffee, tea, or any type of citrus juice before exercising, as these can exacerbate reflux. As part of the Healing Phase, you will be already eliminating these beverages full time, but even after you've completed the initial phase, it's a good pre-exercise rule to follow.

DON'T DO EXERCISES THAT PUT EXCESS STRAIN ON YOUR ABDOMINAL WALL OR ENCOURAGE UPWARD MOVEMENT OF GASTRIC ACID

When it comes to preventing reflux, the type of exercise you do can be just as important a consideration as the timing. Movements that require intense strain of the abdominal wall, which is essentially your core, should be avoided, as should those that require a sustained crouched position and others that repeatedly put your head below your waist. These include the following:

- Heavy weight lifting
- Sit-ups, crunches, leg lifts, and similar abdominal exercises (though a properly done "plank" exercise may be well tolerated)
- Competitive cycling, which would require a crouched position. (Spin classes can require a similar position, but in most cases you should be able to adjust the handlebar height so you are not overly crouched.)
- Gymnastics or advanced yoga

- Any activity that requires excessive jumping—high-impact aerobics, vigorous running, jumping rope
- Surfing, which places extended pressure on the upper abdomen

If you already engage in these activities regularly, it doesn't necessarily mean you should stop what you're doing. But you should pay special attention to the rule about meal timing and when to exercise. Be strict about letting two to three hours pass before exercising and make note of any change in your symptoms. If you find that any activity triggers reflux flare-ups, stop doing it until you've completed the Healing Phase.

Some reflux-safe exercises you can try include cycling, done on a stationary bike or one with handles that don't require an overly crouched position; brisk walking; gentle yoga; strength training (no heavy weights); and bodyweight training with short bouts of moderate to vigorous activity. Extended periods of vigorous exercise can exacerbate acid reflux and increase inflammation, so aim to keep all-out segments on the shorter side. Again, the most important part of exercising with reflux is to pay attention to how you feel. Tolerance for exercise will vary from person to person for movement, and you may find that making adjustments in when you eat relative to when you exercise makes all the difference.

DON'T DRINK SPORTS DRINKS DURING OR AFTER EXERCISE (OR EVER, REALLY)

Many sports drinks, especially Gatorade, contain high amounts of citric acid, which can directly damage your esophageal tissue. You shouldn't drink these types of beverages at all if you're dealing with acid reflux, but especially not when you're exercising and there could already be increased pressure on your LES.

When You're Ready: A HIIT Workout for Your Health

High-intensity interval training (HIIT) is a style of training that's caught on over the last few years, thanks in large part to its short and efficient workouts. This type of training will typically have you perform bodyweight exercises at alternating intensities, from all-out to little to no effort, and workouts can be as short as seven minutes and as long as forty-five. The benefits to HIIT are many: it can be one of the most effective ways to change body composition and burn abdominal fat; it can also help improve endothelial function, which is important to circulation and cellular functions throughout the body, including in the esophagus; and it is highly effective at improving glucose control, which will help you maintain balanced blood sugar. And perhaps the best part of all—it is completely customizable to your fitness level. You can determine exactly what a vigorous effort means for you.

I've seen interval training help many people change their bodies, if only because it helps eliminate the excuse of not having time to work out. That was my personal experience with the HIIT workouts I've completed—although it's tough, you can break a solid sweat and be done and showering, all within forty minutes.

You can try the beginner HIIT workouts offered here, which I've created in collaboration with Faith Murphy, a New York City–based fitness instructor who is certified by the National Academy of Sports Medicine and the International Sports Sciences Association, as well as the elite Equinox fitness club. Because of the more intense intervals, you will want to get a warm-up in before you start any HIIT workout; cold muscles don't usually respond well to an all-out effort, no matter how short. Then, complete one of the three workouts offered—one is cardio on a stationary bike, one is cardio with running or walking, and the other is based on bodyweight exercises. Whichever one you choose, be sure to monitor your reflux symptoms and modify the intensity as needed.

HIIT WARM-UP
Complete as many rounds possible in 5 minutes without stopping

Beginner

Activity	Repetitions
Air squat	10
Jumping jack	20
Reverse lunge left	5
Reverse lunge right	5
Knee push-up	5
Plank hip opener alternating leg	10
Sit-up	5

HIIT CARDIO BIKE

Beginner—37 Minutes

Minutes	Activity
5 min	Warm-up pedal
1 min	Breathless pedal—Created with either gear, resistance, speed, or combination
3 min	Recovery pedal
1 min	Breathless pedal—Created with either gear, resistance, speed, or combination
3 min	Recovery pedal
1 min	Breathless pedal—Created with either gear, resistance, speed, or combination
3 min	Recovery pedal
1 min	Breathless pedal—Created with either gear, resistance, speed, or combination
3 min	Recovery pedal

1 min	Breathless pedal—Created with either gear, resistance, speed, or combination
3 min	Recovery pedal
1 min	Breathless pedal—Created with either gear, resistance, speed, or combination
3 min	Recovery pedal
3 min	Challenging pedal that can be maintained for 3 minutes
5 min	Cool down—slower pedal

HIIT CARDIO WALK/RUN/SPRINT

Beginner—32 minutes

Minutes	Activity
5 min	Warm-up walk
5 min	Brisk walk
30 sec	Jog
3 min	Walk
30 sec	Jog
3 min	Walk
30 sec	Jog
3 min	Walk
30 sec	Jog
3 min	Walk
1 min	Jog
5 min	Walk—cool down

HIIT BODYWEIGHT AS EXERCISES

Complete as many rounds as possible in 20 minutes, with a 30-to-60-second rest between each completed round.

Beginner	Repetitions/Duration
Burpee Modified— squat, step out to plank, step back to squat, stand	5 sets
Dolphin Shoulder Push-Up— plank, walk feet closer to hands to create V with body, bend elbows, and straighten	5 sets
Reverse Lunge—alternating legs	10 sets
Straight-Arm Plank	30 seconds
Wide Squat—squat low, chest up, hands on hips	10 sets
On Hands and Knees Core Work— extend right arm straight out and return, extend left arm straight out and return	4 sets
On Hands and Knees Core Work— extend left leg straight out and return, extend right leg straight out and return	4 sets

HIIT COOL DOWN AND STRETCH

Cat and Cow

Cat: On hands and knees position; round back and drop head.

Cow: On hands and knees position; drop stomach, chest forward, look up.

Shoulder/Core

Start from hands and knees, lift right arm, twist to left, placing right arm through and under left arm, palm up, right cheek on floor. Return to hands and knees.

Lift left arm, twist to right, placing left arm through and under right arm, palm up, left cheek on floor.

Kneeling Hip Flexor/Hamstring/Quad

Left foot in front, chest up, straight spine, right knee down. Move body forward until stretch is achieved in front of the right leg.

Sit back on right heel, extend left leg straight for hamstring.

Right foot in front, chest up, straight spine, left knee down. Move body forward until stretch is achieved in front of the left leg.

Sit back on left heel, extend right leg straight for hamstring.

Child's Pose

Begin in a kneeling position. Then lower your butt to rest on your heels and hinge forward from your pelvis. Walk your hands in front of you, reaching your arms long and straight. Slowly lower your torso all the way to your thighs and rest your forehead on the floor. Place your head on a block or blanket if it doesn't comfortably come to the ground.

The Final Word on Exercise and Acid Reflux

As a physician interested in your general health and longevity, I am an advocate of you simply getting more movement—no matter what type—into each day. This is especially true if you spend a lot of your day sitting, an activity that has been called the "new smoking" because of its link to an increased risk of certain cancers, heart disease, and type 2 diabetes. The link could have something to do with the fact that sedentary time has been associated with elevated levels of inflammation, which we know has links to a long list of diseases.

Because I am a specialist, my interest is more focused—I want the movement you do to be strategic and to complement the eating plan by helping accelerate your recovery from acid damage. In this case, movement isn't just about exercise but includes how you breathe and how and when you move, particularly after you eat. You know now that the best type of exercise for an Acid Watcher is one that isn't too strenuous, as this can trigger reflux; promotes weight loss, especially in the abdominal region; is customizable based on fitness level; and is something with which you can be consistent. Based on these criteria, I encourage you to try the HIIT workouts introduced in this chapter, but any increases you can make in your daily movement will be better than none at all.

Before you hit the gym or head out the door for your walk, remember this: the most powerful tool against acid reflux will be the dietary changes you've read about in earlier chapters, but exercise can help produce profound improvements beyond those that you might experience by following the diet alone.

Conclusion

LIVING A REFLUX-FREE LIFE

Early in this book, you learned that we are at a critical tipping point with acid-related disease. In the United States alone, more than sixty million people experience GERD at least once a month, and each day forty-six people are diagnosed with esophageal cancer, the most severe manifestation of acid damage. I hope you're now walking away with an understanding that acid damage and its associated diseases are not inevitable, and that you, as a newly graduated Acid Watcher, are hereby empowered to reverse the trend toward more severe forms of acid damage. You won't have to do it alone, of course—this bible for survival in a high-acid world will always be with you.

When it's not by your side, you can fall back on the foundational principles of the program, as these will never fail you. To stave off acid damage and the destructive soldiers of inflammation, stay smoke free, eat on time, continue to practice low-acid cooking techniques, and enjoy only minimally processed food. Be sure to eat a diet that consists of low-acid foods balanced with natural macronutrients and micronutrients along with a high-fiber component. And of course, say no to soda.

In my own practice, patients have continued to change their lives by adhering consistently to these principles. Those with heartburn and regurgitation have experienced dramatic and sustainable improvements—so much so that almost everyone who doesn't have a diagnosis of Barrett's esophagus has been able to get off PPIs. The same can be said for the people who have come to me with throatburn reflux symptoms, such as chronic cough, hoarseness, lumplike sensation in the throat, frequent throat clearing, postnasal drip, and difficulty swallowing. In other words: the diet works, if you continue to work it.

The cherry on top (natural, not maraschino, which has been steeped in acid!) has been the response from patients who've also been dealing with autoimmune diseases such as irritable bowel syndrome (IBS), Crohn's disease, psoriasis, fibromyalgia, and rheumatoid arthritis. A strict adherence to the Healing Phase of the Acid Watcher Diet has helped them decrease and, in some cases, eliminate their symptoms and requirements for anti-inflammatory medications such as steroids and nonsteroidal anti-inflammatory drugs (NSAIDs). The anti-inflammatory effect of the diet, it seemed, was profound enough to cool inflammation throughout the body. But this was just a theory until the very day I was wrapping up the writing of this book, when a game-changing study was published in the *Journal of the American Medical Association*.

This study, published on May 17, 2016, and the corresponding editorial, provided proof that refluxed acid initiates a deep-tissue inflammatory response, which sets off the release of a multiplying body of pro-inflammatory proteins. The link between acid damage and worsening systemic inflammatory symptoms, which I had witnessed in practice for so many years, had essentially been scientifically validated.

It's difficult to overstate the clinical significance of this finding, but it's simple to tell you what this means to you and your (hopefully) enduring commitment to a low-acid diet: the payoff is likely to extend far beyond the elimination of your reflux symptoms and could ultimately translate to a lower risk for many of the so-called diseases of inflammation that plague so many people today.

Your larger lifestyle also plays a role in keeping acid damage and inflammation at bay, but you shouldn't overthink it. Aim to exercise often because it will help promote healthy weight, better sleep, and a greater tolerance for stress (and remember: the more consistent your physical activity habit, the more enjoyment and the greater your results). Practice breathing techniques that will create feelings of calm even in the midst of a stressful day and learn to use these in the evenings, too, when drifting off into dreamland is difficult.

Passing the Throatburn Torch

If I could leave you with one final, vital point, it would be to request a carrying of the throatburn torch. You are now in possession of powerful information—the knowledge that throat symptoms such as cough, hoarseness, throat clearing, and a lumplike sensation in the throat can indicate the presence of prolonged acid damage, the type that precedes what is likely to become the second most common form of cancer in the United States, esophageal cancer. Spreading this extremely important message has become my personal crusade, and one that I intend to continue until the perception that acid reflux is innocuous changes. I hope that as a part of the informed minority, you will help me spread this message.

This is not to say you should be passing out anything resembling a diagnosis, but I do hope you will encourage anyone you know with ongoing throat-centered symptoms to visit their doctor, or even to pick up *The Acid Watcher Diet* as a starting point. My ultimate hope is that we can stop esophageal cancer's rising trend and begin to ultimately reverse its course. We can only accomplish this together.

Low-Acid Menus for Special Occasions

Although feeding and entertaining larger groups of people may seem challenging for an Acid Watcher, there are still plenty of options that you and your guests can enjoy. The best part is that no one will even notice that some of the ubiquitous acid-inducing ingredients are gone. And once you are in the Maintenance Phase, you can get really creative. Just multiply the ingredients for the number of people attending and go with the recipes in this book. Consider these options for special occasions:

Valentine's Day Dinner for Two

Roasted Beets and Fresh Cucumber with Creamy White Bean Dip (page 182)

Miso-Agave-Glazed Halibut with Sesame Bok Choy (page 174)

Luxurious "Chocolate" Torte (page 236)

Weekend Brunch

Fresh fruit platter

A platter of "mezze" dips—Apple-Beet Tapenade (page 209), Olive-Artichoke Pâté (page 210), and Lima Bean "Faux" Hummus (page 211) with raw vegetables

Goat Cheese and Spinach Frittata (page 207)

Coconut-Carrot Bars (page 239)

Zucchini Muffins with "Chocolate" Ganache (page 241)

Summer Barbecue

Roasted and Fresh Vegetable GAWzpacho (page 216)

Mexican Shrimp Salad with Avocado, Black Beans, and Cilantro (page 179)

Turkey Burgers with Arugula-Ginger Salad (page 175)

Watermelon Mozzarella Cocktail (page 187)

Acid Watcher Chunky Monkey Cookies (page 232)

Thanksgiving Day Feast

Puréed Butternut Squash Soup with Seared Mushrooms and Herbs (page 184)

Lean and Mean Cottage Pie (page 222)

Brussels Sprout Salad with Pecans, Raisins, and Apple (page 228)

After-dinner cheese plate

Apple Crostata (page 234)

New Year's Day Party

Wild Mushroom Barley Soup (page 218)

Beet and Quinoa Salad with Steamed Kale and Chickpeas (page 183)

Stuffed Baked Salmon with Sweet Potato (page 213)

Poached Pears with Carob Ganache and Pistachios (page 191)

Additional Reading

I encourage you to continue learning more about the latest news about acid reflux disease and updates on research and the latest discoveries at my website, acidwatcher.com. If you are interested in the clinical literature on the subject, I encourage you to look up the studies listed in the Sources section of the book. If you are interested in expanding your knowledge about the food industry, the dietary challenges we are facing, what the future might look like, and what you can do about it, I recommend the following books:

Food Matters: A Guide to Conscious Eating by Mark Bittman. New York: Simon and Schuster, 2009.

Bitter Harvest: A Chef's Perspective on the Hidden Dangers in the Foods We Eat and What You Can Do about It by Ann Cooper and Lisa M. Holmes. New York: Routledge, 2000.

Salt Sugar Fat: How the Food Giants Hooked Us by Michael Moss. New York: Random House, 2014.

The Omnivore's Dilemma: A Natural History of Four Meals by Michael Pollan. New York: Penguin, 2006.

Sources

Additional resources for the *Acid Watcher Diet* can be found at acid watcher.com.

Introduction

Nason, K, P Wichienkuer et al. "Gastroesophageal Reflux Disease Symptom Severity, Proton Pump Inhibitor Use, and Esophageal Carcinogenesis." *Archives of Surgery* 146, no. 7 (2011): 851–858.

Siegel, RL, KD Miller et al. "Cancer Statistics, 2016." *CA: A Cancer Journal for Clinicians* 66, no. 1 (2016): 7–30.

Chapter 1: Dietary Acid Damage

Dent J, HB El-Serag et al. "Epidemiology of Gastro-Oesophageal Reflux Disease: A Systematic Review." *Gut* 54, no. 5 (2005): 710–717.

El-Serag, HB, S Sweet et al. "Update on the Epidemiology of Gastro-Oesophageal Reflux Disease: A Systematic Review." *Gut* 63, no. 6 (2014): 871–880.

Fass R, SF Quan et al. "Predictors of Heartburn during Sleep in a Large Prospective Cohort Study." *Chest* 127, no. 5 (2005): 1658–1666.

Koufman, JA. "Low-Acid Diet for Recalcitrant Laryngopharyngeal Reflux: Therapeutic Benefits and Their Implications." *Annals of Otology, Rhinology and Laryngology* 120, no. 5 (2011): 281–287.

Koufman, JA, JE Aviv et al. "Laryngopharyngeal Reflux: Position Statement of the Committee on Speech, Voice, and Swallowing Disorders of the American Academy of Otolaryngology–Head and Neck Surgery." *Otolaryngology Head and Neck Surgery* 127, no. 1 (2002): 32–35.

Niemantsverdriet, EC, R Timmer et al. "The Roles of Excessive Gastrooesophageal Reflux, Disordered Oesophageal Motility and Decreased Mucosal Sensitivity in the Pathogenesis of Barrett's Oesophagus." *European Journal of Gastroenterology and Hepatology* 9, no. 5 (1997): 515–519.

Reavis, K, C Morris et al. "Laryngopharyngeal Reflux Symptoms Better Predict the Presence of Esophageal Adenocarcinoma Than Typical Gastroesophageal Reflux Symptoms." *Annals of Surgery* 239, no. 6 (2004): 849–858.

Chapter 2: Acid Reflux, Your Esophagus, and the Cancer Connection

Angelopoulos, TJ, J Lowndes et al. "The Effect of High-Fructose Corn Syrup Consumption on Triglycerides and Uric Acid." *Journal of Nutrition* 139, no. 6 (2009): 1242S–1245S.

Aviv, JE. "pH Basics and the pH of Commonly Consumed Foods." In *Killing Me Softly from Inside: The Mysteries and Dangers of Acid Reflux and Its Connection to America's Fastest Growing Cancer with a Diet That May Save Your Life,* 70–78. North Charleston, SC: CreateSpace, 2014.

Carpenter, M. "Introduction: A Bitter White Powder." In *Caffeinated: How Our Daily Habit Helps, Hurts and Hooks Us,* xvi. New York: Hudson Street Press, 2014.

———. "Why Do Americans Drink Half as Much Coffee Today as They Did 60 Years Ago?" Zócalo Public Square. April 22, 2014. http://www.zocalopublicsquare.org/2014/04/21/why-do-americans-drink-half-as-much-coffee-today-as-they-did-60-years-ago/ideas/nexus/.

Chin, TW, M Loeb et al. "Effects of an Acidic Beverage (Coca-Cola) on Absorption of Ketoconazole." *Antimicrobial Agents and Chemotherapeutics* 39, no. 8 (1995): 1671–1675.

Lacy, BE, J Carter et al. "The Effects of Intraduodenal Nutrient Infusion on Serum CCK, LES Pressure, and Gastroesophageal Reflux." *Neurogastroenterology and Motility* 23, no. 7 (2011): 631–638.

Lada, MJ, DR Nieman et al. "Gastroesophageal Reflux Disease, Proton-Pump Inhibitor Use and Barrett's Esophagus in Esophageal Adenocarcinoma: Trends Revisited." *Surgery* 154, no. 4 (2013): 856–866.

Lyden, E. "High Fructose Corn Syrup: A Food to Completely Avoid to Stay Healthy." Mic. October 6, 2012. http://mic.com/articles/15310/high-fructose-corn-syrup-a-food-to-completely-avoid-to-stay-healthy.

McQuaid, KR, and L Laine. "A Systematic Review and Meta-Analysis of Randomized, Controlled Trials of Moderate Sedation for Routine Endoscopic Procedures." *Gastrointestinal Endoscopy* 67, no. 6 (2008): 910–923.

Moss, M. *Salt Sugar Fat: How the Food Giants Hooked Us.* New York: Random House, 2014.

Peery, AF, ES Dellon et al. "Burden of Gastrointestinal Disease in the United States: 2012 Update." *Gastroenterology* 143, no. 5 (2012): 1179–1187.

Pohl, H, and HG Welch. "The Role of Over-Diagnosis and Reclassification in the Marked Increase of Esophageal Adenocarcinoma Incidence." *Journal of the National Cancer Institute* 97, no. 2 (2004): 142–146.

Samuels, TL, AC Pearson et al. "Curcumin and Anthocyanin Inhibit Pepsin-Mediated Cell Damage and Carcinogenic Changes in Airway Epithelial Cells." *Annals of Otology, Rhinology and Laryngology* 122, no. 10 (2013): 632–641.

Sandner, A, J Illert et al. "Reflux Induces DNA Strand Breaks and Expression Changes of MMP1+9+14 in a Human Miniorgan Culture Model." *Experimental Cell Research* 319, no. 19 (2013): 2905–2915.

Shaheen, NJ, GW Falk et al. "ACG Clinical Guideline: Diagnosis and Management of Barrett's Esophagus." *American Journal of Gastroenterology* 111, no. 1 (2016): 30–50.

Soyer, T, OU Soyer et al. "Pepsin Levels and Oxidative Stress Markers in Exhaled Breath Condensate of Patients with Gastroesophageal Reflux Disease." *Journal of Pediatric Surgery* 48, no. 11 (2013): 2247–2250.

Stanhope, KL, JM Schwarz et al. "Consuming Fructose-Sweetened, Not Glucose-Sweetened, Beverages Increases Visceral Adiposity and Lipids and Decreases Insulin Sensitivity in Overweight/Obese Humans." *Journal of Clinical Investigation* 119, no. 5 (2009): 1322–1334.

U.S. Food and Drug Administration. "Draft Guidance for Industry: Acidified Foods. Food and Drug Administration." Updated January 11, 2016. http://www.fda.gov/Food/GuidanceRegulation/GuidanceDocuments RegulatoryInformation/AcidifiedLACF/default.htm.

Chapter 3: Inflamed

Amara, BI, A Karray et al. "Dimethoate Induces Kidney Dysfunction, Disrupts Membrane-Bound ATPases and Confers Cytotoxicity through DNA Damage: Protective Effects of Vitamin E and Selenium." *Biological Trace Element Research* 156 (2013): 230–242.

Ayzi, S, JA Hagen et al. "Obesity and Gastroesophageal Reflux: Quantifying the Association between Body Mass Index, Esophageal Acid Exposure, and Lower Esophageal Sphincter Status in a Large Series of Patients with Reflux Symptoms." *Journal of Gastrointestinal Surgery* 13 (2009): 1440–1447.

Fisichella, PM, and MG Patti. "Gastroesophageal Reflux Disease and Morbid Obesity: Is There a Relation?" *Société Internationale de Chirurgie* 33 (2009): 2034–2038.

Gorman, C, A Park et al. "Cellular Inflammation: The Secret Killer." Peabody, MA: Inflammation Research Foundation, 2015.

Groopman, J. "Inflamed: The Debate over the Latest Cure-All Craze." *New Yorker.* November 30, 2015. http://www.newyorker.com/magazine/2015/11/30/inflamed.

Huneault, L, ME Mathieu et al. "Globalization and Modernization: An Obesogenic Combination." *Obesity Review* 12 (2011): e64–e72.

Lobo, V, A Patel et al. "Free Radicals, Antioxidants, and Functional Foods: Impact on Human Health." *Pharmacognosy Review* 4, no. 8 (2010): 118–126.

Marseglia, L, G D'Angelo et al. "Oxidative Stress in Obesity: A Critical Component in Human Diseases." *International Journal of Molecular Sciences* 16 (2015): 378–400.

Nutrition Science Initiative. "By the Numbers." Accessed June 20, 2016. http://www.nusi.org/by-the-numbers/.

Priyanka, A, AS Sasidharan et al. "Curcumin Improves Hypoxia Induced Dysfunctions in 3T3-L1 Adipocytes by Protecting Mitochondria and Down Regulating Inflammation." *BioFactors* 40 (2014): 513–523.

Rahman, K. "Studies on Free Radicals, Antioxidants, and Co-Factors." *Clinical Interventions in Aging* 2, no. 2 (2007): 219–236.

Shahteen, N, GW Falk et al. "ACG Clinical Guideline: Diagnosis and Management of Barrett's Esophagus." *American Journal of Gastroenterology* (2015). doi:10.1038/ajg.2015.322.

Chapter 4: Seeking Treatment

Aisenberg J, JV Brill et al. "Sedation for Gastrointestinal Endoscopy: New Practices, New Economics." *American Journal of Gastroenterology* 100, no. 5 (2005): 996–1000.

Al-Awabdy, B, and CM Wilcox. "Use of Anesthesia on the Rise in Gastrointestinal Endoscopy." *World Journal of Gastrointestinal Endoscopy* 16, no. 5 (2013): 1–5.

Altman, K, CB Simpson et al. "Cough and Paradoxical Vocal Fold Motion." *Otolaryngology Head and Neck Surgery* 127, no. 6 (2002): 501–511.

Aviv, JE. "Transnasal Esophagoscopy: State of the Art." *Otolaryngology Head and Neck Surgery* 135, no. 4 (2006): 616–619.

Aviv, JE, T Takoudes et al. "Office-Based Esophagoscopy: A Preliminary Report." *Otolaryngology Head and Neck Surgery* 125, no. 3 (2001): 170–175.

Aviv, JE, and LF Johnson. "Flexible Endoscopic Evaluation of Swallowing with Sensory Testing (FEESST) to Diagnose and Manage Patients with Pharyngeal Dysphagia." *Practical Gastroenterology* 24 (2000): 52–59.

Aviv, JE, M Parides et al. "Endoscopic Evaluation of Swallowing as an Alternative to 24-Hour pH Monitoring to Diagnose Extra-Esophageal Reflux." *Annals of Otology, Rhinology and Laryngology* 109, suppl. 184 (2000): 25–27.

Christopher, KL, RP Wood II et al. "Vocal-Cord Dysfunction Presenting as Asthma." *New England Journal of Medicine* 308, no. 26 (1983): 1566–1570.

Cohen, L, M DeLegge et al. "AGA Institute Review of Endoscopic Sedation." *Gastroenterology* 133, no. 2 (2007): 675–701.

Cohen, LB, and AA Benson. "Issues in Endoscopic Sedation." *Gastroenterology and Hepatology* 5, no. 8 (2009): 565–570.

Enestvedt, BK, GM Eisen et al. "Is the American Society of Anesthesiologists Classification Useful in Risk Stratification for Endoscopic Procedures?" *Gastrointestinal Endoscopy* 77, no. 3 (2013): 464–471.

Harding, SM, and JE Richter. "The Role of Gastroesophageal Reflux in Chronic Cough and Asthma." *Chest* 111, no. 5 (1997): 1389–1402.

Lee, B, and P Woo. "Chronic Cough as a Sign of Laryngeal Sensory Neuropathy: Diagnosis and Treatment." *Annals of Otology, Rhinology and Laryngology* 114, no. 4 (2005): 253–257.

Liu, H, DA Waxman et al. "Utilization of Anesthesia Services during Outpatient Endoscopies and Colonoscopies and Associated Spending in 2003–2009." *Journal of the American Medical Association* 307, no. 11 (2012): 1178–1184.

McQuaid, K, and L Laine. "A Systematic Review and Meta-Analysis of Randomized, Controlled Trials of Moderate Sedation for Routine Endoscopic Procedures." *Gastrointestinal Endoscopy* 67, no. 6 (2008): 910–923.

Mintz, S, and JK Lee. "Gabapentin in the Treatment of Intractable Chronic Cough: Case Reports." *American Journal of Medicine* 119, no. 5 (2006): 13–15.

Mishriki, YY. "Laryngeal Neuropathy as a Cause of Chronic Intractable Cough." *American Journal of Medicine* 120, no. 2 (2007): 5–7.

Morrison, M, L Rammage et al. "The Irritable Larynx Syndrome." *Journal of Voice* 13, no. 3 (1999): 447–455.

Murry, T, R Branski et al. "Laryngeal Sensory Deficits in Patients with Chronic Cough and Paradoxical Vocal Fold Movement Disorder." *Laryngoscope* 120, no. 8 (2010): 1576–1581.

Murry, T, and C Sapienza. "The Role of Voice Therapy in the Management of Paradoxical Vocal Fold Motion, Chronic Cough, and Laryngospasm." *Otolaryngology Clinics of North America* 43, no. 1 (2010): 73–83.

Murry, T, A Tabaee et al. "Respiratory Retraining of Refractory Cough and Laryngopharyngeal Reflux in Patients with Paradoxical Vocal Fold Movement Disorder." *Laryngoscope* 114, no. 8 (2004): 1341–1345.

Murry, T, A Tabaee et al. "Respiratory Retraining Therapy and Management of Laryngopharyngeal Reflux in the Treatment of Patients with Cough and Paradoxical Vocal Fold Movement Disorder." *Annals of Otology, Rhinology and Laryngology* 115, no. 10 (2006): 754–758.

Newman, KB, UG Mason III et al. "Clinical Features of Vocal Cord Dysfunction." *American Journal of Respiratory and Critical Care Medicine* 152, no. 4 (1995): 1382–1386.

Petrini, J, and J Egan. "Risk Management Regarding Sedation/Analgesia." *Gastrointestinal Endoscopic Clinicians of North America* 14, no. 2 (2004): 401–414.

Phua, SY, LP McGarvey et al. "Patients with Gastro-Esophageal Reflux Disease and Cough Have Impaired Laryngopharyngeal Mechanosensitivity." *Thorax* 60, no. 6: 488–491.

Rex, DK, VP Deenadayalu et al. "Endoscopist-Directed Administration of Propofol: A Worldwide Safety Experience." *Gastroenterology* 137, no. 4 (2009): 1229–1237.

Rogers, JH, and PM Stell. "Paradoxical Movement of the Vocal Cords as a Cause of Stridor." *Journal of Laryngology and Otology* 92, no. 2 (1978): 157–158.

U.S. Preventive Services Task Force. "Screening for Colorectal Cancer: U.S. Preventive Services Task Force Recommendation Statement." AHRQ Publication 08-05124-EF-3. Rockville, MD: Agency for Healthcare Research and Quality, 2008.

Vargo, JJ, LB Cohen et al. "Position Statement: Nonanesthesiologist Administration of Propofol for GI Endoscopy." *American Journal of Gastroenterology* 104, no. 12 (2009): 2886–2892.

Vertigan, AE, DG Theodoros et al. "The Relationship between Chronic Cough and Paradoxical Vocal Fold Movement: A Review of the Literature." *Journal of Voice* 20, no. 3 (2006): 466–480.

Wani, MK, and GE Woodson. "Paroxysmal Laryngospasm after Laryngeal Nerve Injury." *Laryngoscope* 109, no. 5 (1999): 694–697.

Chapter 5: Understanding the Role of Proteins, Carbohydrates, and Fats in Healing Dietary Acid Damage

Basson, M. "Gut Mucosal Healing: Is the Science Relevant?" *American Journal of Pathology* 161, no 4 (2002): 1101–1105.

Berry, W, and M Pollan. *Bringing It to the Table: On Farming and Food.* Berkeley, CA: Counterpoint Press, 2009.

Donaghue, K, M Pena et al. "Beneficial Effects of Increasing Monounsaturated Fat Intake in Adolescents with Type 1 Diabetes." *Diabetes Research and Clinical Practice* 48, no. 3 (2000): 193–199.

Dukan, P. *The Dukan Diet: 2 Steps to Lose the Weight, 2 Steps to Keep It Off Forever.* New York: Crown, 2011.

El-Serag, H, J Satia et al. "Dietary Intake and the Risk of Gastro-Esophageal Reflux Disease: A Cross Sectional Study in Volunteers." *Gut* 54, no. 1 (2005): 11–17.

Esselstyn, C. *Prevent and Reverse Heart Disease: The Revolutionary, Scientifically Proven, Nutrition-Based Cure.* New York: Penguin, 2007.

Food and Nutrition Board, Institute of Medicine of the National Academies. "Dietary Reference Intakes for Energy, Carbohydrate, Fiber, Fat, Fatty Acids, Cholesterol, Protein, and Amino Acids." Washington, DC: National Academies Press, 2005.

Gates, D, and L Schrecengost. *The Baby Boomer Diet: Body Ecology's Guide to Growing Younger.* Carlsbad, CA: Hay House, 2011.

Hernandez-Alonse, P, J Salas-Salvado et al. "High Dietary Protein Intake Is Associated with an Increased Body Weight and Total Death Risk." *Clinical Nutrition* 35, no. 2 (2016): 496–506.

Rybicki, S. "The Importance of HUFAs in Fish Food." Accessed June 20, 2016. http://www.angelsplus.com/ArticleHufa.htm.

Savarino, E, N de Bortoli et al. "Alginate Controls Heartburn in Patients with Erosive and Nonerosive Reflux Disease." *World Journal of Gastroenterology* 18, no. 32 (2012): 4371–4378.

Simopoulos, A. "The Importance of the Omega-6/Omega-3 Fatty Acid Ratio in Cardiovascular Disease and Other Chronic Diseases." *Experimental Biology and Medicine* 233, no. 6 (2008): 674–688.

Taubes, G. "What If It's All Been a Big Fat Lie?" *New York Times,* July 7, 2007. http://www.nytimes.com/2002/07/07/magazine/what-if-it-s-all-been-a-big-fat-lie.html?pagewanted=all&src=pm.

Watson, B, and L Smith. *The Fiber35 Diet: Nature's Weight Loss Secret.* New York: Free Press, 2007.

Chapter 6: The Fiber Gap and How to Bridge It

de Koning, L, and FB Hu. "Do the Health Benefits of Dietary Fiber Extend beyond Cardiovascular Disease?" *Archives of Internal Medicine* 171, no. 12 (2011): 1069–1070.

Ghanim, H, M Batra et al. "The Intake of Fiber Suppresses the High Fat High Carbohydrate Meal Induced Endotoxemia, Oxidative Stress and Inflammation." *Endocrine Abstracts* 29 (2012): 613.

Lattimer, JM, and MD Haub. "Effects of Dietary Fiber and Its Components on Metabolic Health." *Nutrients* 2, no. 12 (2010): 1266–1289.

Ma, Y, JA Griffith et al. "Association between Dietary Fiber and Serum C-Reactive Protein." *American Journal of Clinical Nutrition* 83, no. 4 (2006): 760–766.

Park, Y, AF Subar et al. "Dietary Fiber Intake and Mortality in the NIH-AARP Diet and Health Study." *Archives of Internal Medicine* 171, no. 12 (2011): 1061–1068.

Pereira, MA, E O'Reilly et al. "Dietary Fiber and Risk of Coronary Heart Disease: A Pooled Analysis of Cohort Studies." *Archives of Internal Medicine* 164, no. 4 (2004): 370–376.

Rao, SSC, S Yu et al. "Dietary Fibre and FODMAP-Restricted Diet in the Management of Constipation and Irritable Bowel Syndrome." *Alimentary Pharmacology and Therapeutics* 41, no. 12 (2015): 1256–1270.

Slavin, JL. "Position of the American Dietetic Association: Health Implications of Dietary Fiber." *Journal of the American Dietetic Association* 108, no. 10 (2008): 1716–1731.

Threapleton, DE, DC Greenwood et al. "Dietary Fibre Intake and Risk of Cardiovascular Disease: Systematic Review and Meta-Analysis." *British Medical Journal* 347 (2013): f6879.

Watson, B, and L Smith. *The Fiber35 Diet: Nature's Weight Loss Secret.* New York: Free Press, 2007.

Chapter 7: Developing Your pH Savvy

Bonjour, JP. "Nutritional Disturbance in Acid Base Balance and Osteoporosis: A Hypothesis That Disregards the Essential Homeostatic Role of the Kidney." *British Journal of Nutrition* 110 (2013): 1168–1177.

Chiva-Blanch, G, L Badimon et al. "Latest Evidence of the Effects of the Mediterranean Diet in Prevention of Cardiovascular Disease." *Current Atherosclerosis Reports* 16, no. 10 (2014): 446.

Dwyer, J, E Foulkes et al. "Acid/Alkaline Ash Diets: Time for Assessment and Change." *Journal of the American Dietetic Association* 85, no. 7 (1985): 841–845.

Fenton, TR, AW Lyon et al. "Meta-Analysis of the Effect of the Acid-Ash Hypothesis of Osteoporosis on Calcium Balance." *Journal of Bone and Mineral Research* 24, no. 11 (2009): 1835–1840.

Frassetto, L, R Morris et al. "Diet, Evolution and Aging: The Pathophysiologic Effects of the Post-Agricultural Inversion of the Potassium-to-Sodium and Base-to-Chloride Ratios in the Human Diet." *European Journal of Nutrition* 40, no. 5 (2001): 200–213.

Fung, T, FB Hu et al. "The Mediterranean and Dietary Approaches to Stop Hypertension Diets and Colorectal Cancer." *American Journal of Clinical Nutrition* 92, no. 6 (2010): 1429–1435.

Hernandez-Alonse, P, J Salas-Salvado et al. "High Dietary Protein Intake Is Associated with an Increased Body Weight and Total Death Risk." *Clinical Nutrition* 35, no. 2 (2016): 496–506.

Johnston, N, P Dettmar et al. "Activity/Stability of Human Pepsin: Implications for Reflux Attributed Laryngeal Disease." *Laryngoscope* 117, no. 6 (2007): 1036–1039.

Johnston, N, J Knight et al. "Pepsin and Carbonic Anhydrase Isoenzyme III as Diagnostic Markers for Laryngopharyngeal Reflux Disease." *Laryngoscope* 114, no. 12 (2004): 2129–2134.

Koeppen, BM. "The Kidney and Acid-Base Regulation." *Advances in Physiology Education* 33, no. 4 (2009): 275–281.

Myers, R. "One Hundred Years of pH." *Journal of Chemical Education* 87, no. 1 (2010): 30–32.

Remer, T. "Influence of Diet on Acid-Base Balance." *Seminars in Dialysis* 13, no. 4 (2000): 221–226.

Schwalfenberg, G. "The Alkaline Diet: Is There Evidence That an Alkaline pH Diet Benefits Health?" *Journal of Environmental and Public Health* (2012). Article ID 727630. doi:10.1155/2012/727630.

Speakman, JR, and SE Mitchell. "Caloric Restriction." *Molecular Aspects of Medicine* 32, no. 3 (2011): 159–221.

Tobey, JA. "The Question of Acid and Alkali Forming Foods." *American Journal of Public Health* 26 (1936): 1113–1116.

Tucker, KL, MT Hannan et al. "The Acid-Base Hypothesis: Diet and Bone in the Framingham Osteoporosis Study." *European Journal of Nutrition* 40 (2001): 231–237.

Vyas, B, and S Le Quesne. *The pH Balance Diet: Restore Your Acid-Alkaline Levels to Eliminate Toxins and Lose Weight.* Berkeley, CA: Ulysses Press, 2007.

Young, R, and S Young. *The pH Miracle for Weight Loss: Balance Your Body Chemistry, Achieve Your Ideal Weight.* New York: Hachette, 2010.

Chapter 8: Breaking Acid-Generating Habits and Establishing Acid-Reduction Practices

Bjornholm, M. "Chronic Glucocorticoid Treatment Increases De Novo Lipogenesis in Visceral Adipose Tissue." *Acta Physiologica* 211, no. 2 (2014): 257–259.

Blanaru, M, B Bloch et al. "The Effects of Music Relaxation and Muscle Relaxation Techniques on Sleep Quality and Emotional Measures among Individuals with Post-Traumatic Stress Disorder." *Mental Illness* 4, no. 2 (2012): e13.

Chow, T. "Wake Up and Smell the Coffee: Caffeine, Coffee and the Medical Consequences." *Western Journal of Medicine* 157, no. 5 (1992): 544–553.

Di Carlo, G, and IA Angelo. "Cannabinoids for Gastrointestinal Diseases: Potential Therapeutic Applications." *Expert Opinion on Investigational Drugs* 12, no. 1 (2003): 39–49.

Dua, KS, SN Surapaneni et al. "Effect of Systemic Alcohol and Nicotine on Airway Protective Reflexes." *American Journal of Gastroenterology* 104, no. 10 (2009): 2431–2438.

Gates, P, A Jaffe et al. "Cannabis Smoking and Respiratory Health: Consideration of the Literature." *Respirology* 19, no. 5 (2014): 655–662.

Hall, W. "What Has Research over the Past Two Decades Revealed about the Adverse Health Effects of Recreational Cannabis Use?" *Addiction* 110, no. 1 (2015): 19–35.

Herring, MP, CE Kline et al. "Effects of Exercise on Sleep among Young Women with Generalized Anxiety Disorder." *Mental Health and Physical Activity* 9 (2015): 59–66.

Huang, JY-H, Z-F Zhang et al. "An Epidemologic Review of Marijuana and Cancer: An Update." *Cancer Epidemiology, Biomarkers and Prevention* 24, no. 1 (2015): 15–31.

Huneault, L, ME Mathieu et al. "Globalization and Modernization: An Obesogenic Combination." *Obesity Review* 12 (2011): e64–e72.

Kempker, JA, EG Honig et al. "Effects of Marijuana Exposure on Expiratory Airflow." *Annals of the American Thoracic Society* 12, no. 2 (2014): 135–141.

Konturek, PC, T Brzozowski et al. "Stress and the Gut: Pathophysiology, Clinical Consequences, Diagnostic Approach and Treatment Options." *Journal of Physiology and Pharmacology* 62, no. 6 (2011): 591–599.

Larun, L, KF Brurburg et al. "Exercise Therapy for Chronic Fatigue Syndrome." *Cochrane Database of Systematic Reviews* 10, no. 2 (2015). doi:10.1002/14651858.

Lohsiriwat, S, N Puengna et al. "Effect of Caffeine on Lower Esophageal Sphincter Pressure in Thai Healthy Volunteers." *Diseases of the Esophagus* 19, no. 3 (2006): 183–188.

Lubin, JH, MB Cook et al. "The Importance of Exposure Rate on Odds Ratios by Cigarette Smoking and Alcohol Consumption for Esophageal Adenocarcinoma and Squamous Cell Carcinoma in the Barrett's Esophagus and Esophageal Adenocarcinoma Consortium." *International Journal of Cancer Epidemiology, Detection, and Prevention* 36 (2012): 306–316.

Rasheed, N, and A Alghasham. "Central Dopaminergic System and Its Implications in Stress-Mediated Neurological Disorders and Gastric Ulcers: Short Review." *Advances in Pharmacological Sciences* (2012). Article ID 182671, 11 pages. doi:10.1155/2012/182671.

Rosmond, R, MF Dallman et al. "Stress-Related Cortisol Secretion in Men: Relationships with Abnormal Obesity and Endocrine Metabolic and Hemodynamic Abnormalities." *Journal of Clinical Endocrinology and Metabolism* 83, no. 6 (1998): 1853–1859.

Sansone, RA, and LA Sansone. "Marijuana and Body Weight." *Innovations in Clinical Neuroscience* 11, no. 7/8 (2014): 50–54.

Sharif, F, M Seddigh et al. "The Effect of Aerobic Exercise on Quantity and Quality of Sleep among Elderly People Referring to Health Centers of Lar City, Southern of Iran; A Randomized Controlled Clinical Trial." *Current Aging Science* 8, no. 3 (2015): 248–255.

Stice, E, DP Figlewicz et al. "The Contribution of Brain Reward Circuits to the Obesity Epidemic." *Neuroscience and Biobehavioral Reviews* 37, no. 9 (2013): 2047–2058.

Tojo, R, A Suarez et al. "Intestinal Microbiota in Health and Disease: Role of Bifidobacteria in Gut Homeostasis." *World Journal of Gastroenterology* 20, no. 41 (2014): 15163–15176.

Zhang, Z-F, H Morgenstern et al. "Marijuana Use and Increased Rise of Squamous Cell Carcinoma of the Head and Neck." *Cancer Epidemiology, Biomarkers and Prevention* 8, no. 2 (1999): 1071–1078.

Chapter 9: The Healing Phase (Days 1 to 28)

Amerman, D. "Health Benefits of Star Anise." SFGate. Accessed June 20, 2016. http://www.healthyeatings.sfgate.com.health-benefits-star-anise4835.html.

"Asafoetida: Uses, Side Effects, Interactions and Warnings." WebMD. Accessed June 20, 2016. http://www.webmd.com/vitamins-supplements/ingredientmono-248-asafoetida.aspx.

Aviv, JE, H Liu et al. "Laryngopharyngeal Sensory Deficits in Patients with Laryngopharyngeal Reflux and Dysphagia." *Annals of Otology, Rhinology and Laryngology* 109 (2000): 1000–1006.

Bharat, B, B Aggarwal et al. "Identification of Novel Anti-Inflammatory Agents from Ayurvedic Medicine for Prevention of Chronic Diseases: 'Reverse Pharmacology' and 'Bedside to Bench' Approach." *Current Drug Targets* 12, no. 11 (2011): 1595–1653.

Campbell, TM, and TC Campbell. *The China Study: The Most Comprehensive Study of Nutrition Ever Conducted and the Startling Implications for Diet, Weight Loss and Long-Term Health.* Dallas, TX: BenBella Books, 2004.

"Carob: Better Than Chocolate." Gilead Institute of America. Accessed June 20, 2016. http://www.gilead.net/health/carob.html.

Chung, MY, TG Lim et al. "Molecular Mechanisms of Chemopreventive Phytochemicals against Gastroenterological Cancer Development." *World Journal of Gastroenterology* 19, no. 7 (2013): 984–993.

Coleman, HG, LJ Murray et al. "Dietary Fiber and the Risk of Precancerous Lesions and Cancer of the Esophagus: A Systematic Review and Meta-Analysis." *Nutrition Reviews* 1, no. 7 (2013): 474–482.

"The Healing Effects of Cloves." Global Healing Center. http://www.globalhealingcenter.com/natural-health/health-benefits-of-cloves/

"Health Benefits of Fennel." Organic Facts. Accessed June 20, 2016. https://www.organicfacts.net/health-benefits/herb-and-spices/health-benefits-of-fennel.html.

Hyman, M. "Milk Is Dangerous for Your Health." DrHyman.com. Accessed June 20, 2016. http://drhyman.com/blog/2013/10/28/milk-dangerous-health/.

Kubo, A, TR Levin et al. "Dietary Antioxidants, Fruits, and Vegetables and the Risk of Barrett's Esophagus." *American Journal of Gastroenterology* 103, no. 7 (2008): 1614–1623.

Lustig, RH. *Fat Chance: Beating the Odds against Sugar, Processed Food, Obesity, and Disease.* New York: Hudson Street Press, 2013.

Massey, BT. "Diffuse Esophageal Spasm: A Case for Carminatives?" *Journal of Clinical Gastroenterology* 33, no. 1 (2001): 8–10.

Parker, H. "A Sweet Problem: Princeton Researchers Find That High-Fructose Corn Syrup Prompts Considerably More Weight Gain." March 22, 2010. http://www.princeton.edu/main/news/archive/S26/91/22K07/.

Pollan, M. *In Defense of Food: An Eater's Manifesto.* New York: Penguin, 2008.

Subramanian, S. "Fact or Fiction: Raw Veggies Are Healthier than Cooked Ones." *Scientific American.* March 31, 2009. http://www.scientificamerican.com/articles/raw-veggies-are-healthier/.

"Sumac." TheSpiceHouse.com. http://www.thespicehouse.com/spices/powdered-sumac.

"10 Benefits of Celtic Sea Salt and Himalayan Salt." DrAxe.com. https://draxe.com/10-benefits-celtic-sea-salt-himalayan-salt/.

"Top 10 Foods Highest in Lycopene." HealthAliciousNess.com. Accessed June 20, 2016. http://www.healthaliciousness.com/articles/high-lycopene-foods.php.

Wang, X, and Y Ouyant. "Fruit and Vegetable Consumption and Mortality from All Causes, Cardiovascular Disease, and Cancer: Systematic Review and Dose-Response Meta-Analysis of Prospective Cohort Studies." *British Medical Journal* 349 (2014): g4490. doi:10.1135/bmj.g4490.

"Watermelon Beats Tomatoes in Lycopene Stakes." NutraIngredients-USA.com. June 5, 2002. http://www.nutraingredients-usa.com/Research/Watermelon-beats-tomatoes-in-lycopene-stakes.

Watson, B, and L Smith. *The Fiber35 Diet: Nature's Weight Loss Secret.* New York: Free Press, 2007.

Chapter 10: The Healing Phase
Meal Planner with Recipes

U.S. Food and Drug Administration. "Approximate pH of Foods and Food Products." April 2007. http://www.foodscience.caes.uga.edu/extension/documents/fdaapproximatephoffoodslacf-phs.pdf.

Weil, A. "Cooking with Grains: Buckwheat." DrWeil.com. http://www.drweil.com/drw/u/ART03180/How-to-Cook-Buckwheat-Kasha.html.

Chapter 11: The Maintenance Phase
Meal Planner with Recipes

U.S. Food and Drug Administration. "Approximate pH of Foods and Food Products." April 2007. http://www.foodscience.caes.uga.edu/extension/documents/fdaapproximatephoffoodslacf-phs.pdf.

Chapter 12: Getting pHit

Aronne, LJ, and KR Segal. "Adiposity and Fat Distribution Outcome Measures: Assessment and Clinical Implications." *Obesity Research* 10, no. S11 (2002): 14S–21S.

Colberg, SR, L Zarrabi et al. "Postprandial Walking Is Better for Lowering the Glycemic Effect of Dinner Than Pre-Dinner Exercise in Type 2 Diabetic Individuals." *Journal of the American Medical Directors Association* 10, no. 6 (2009): 394–397.

Després, JP, I Lemieux et al. "Treatment of Obesity: Need to Focus on High Risk Abdominally Obese Patients." *British Medical Journal* 322 (2001): 716–720.

Eherer, AJ, and F Netolitzky. "Positive Effect of Abdominal Breathing Exercise on Gastroesophageal Reflux Disease: A Randomized, Controlled Study." *American Journal of Gastroenterology* 107, no. 3 (2012): 372–378.

Hirshkowitz, M. "How Does Exercise Affect Sleep Duration and Quality?" National Sleep Foundation. February 25, 2013. https://sleepfoundation.org/ask-the-expert/how-does-exercise-affect-sleep-duration-and-quality.

Hoyo, C, MB Cook et al. "Body Mass Index in Relation to Oesophageal and Oesophagogastric Junction Adenocarcinomas: A Pooled Analysis from the International BEACON Consortium." *International Journal of Epidemiology* 41, no. 6 (2012): 1706–1718.

Kashine, S, K Kishida et al. "Selective Contribution of Waist Circumference Reduction on the Improvement of Sleep-Disordered Breathing in Patients Hospitalized with Type 2 Diabetes Mellitus." *Internal Medicine* 50, no. 18 (2011): 1895–1903.

Kwong, MF, and J Khoo. "Diet and Exercise in Management of Obesity and Overweight." *Journal of Gastroenterology and Hepatology* 28, no. S4 (2013): 59–63.

Loprinzia, PD, and BJ Cardinal. "Association between Objectively-Measured Physical Activity and Sleep, NHANES 2005–2006." *Mental Health and Physical Activity* 4, no. 2 (2011): 65–69.

Murao, T, and K Sakurai. "Lifestyle Change Influences on GERD in Japan: A Study of Participants in a Health Examination Program." *Digestive Diseases and Sciences* 56, no. 10 (2011): 2857–2864.

Siddharth, S, D Swapna et al. "Physical Activity Is Associated with Reduced Risk of Esophageal Cancer, Particularly Esophageal Adenocarcinoma: A Systematic Review and Meta-Analysis." *BMC Gastroenterology* 14 (2014). doi:10.1186/1471-230X-14-101.

Song, Q, J Wang et al. "Shorter Dinner-to-Bed Time Is Associated with Gastric Cardia Adenocarcinoma Risk Partly in a Reflux-Dependent Manner." *Annals of Surgical Oncology* 21, no. 8 (2014): 2615–2619.

Conclusion

Dunbar, KB, TA Agoston et al. "Association of Acute Gastroesophageal Reflux Disease with Esophageal Histologic Changes." *Journal of the American Medical Association* 315, no. 19 (2016): 2104.

Kahrilas, PJ. "Turning the Pathogenesis of Acute Peptic Esophagitis Inside Out." *Journal of the American Medical Association* 315, no. 19 (2016): 2077–2078.

Acknowledgments

Just as a surgeon cannot perform an operation alone, no book is ever completed by a single individual.

Thank you to my literary agent, Steve Troha from Folio Lit, who helped me assemble a stellar team. A special thank-you to Gretchen Lees and Julia Serebrinsky for their countless hours of editing, inspiration, and insight. Thank you as well to Diana Baroni and Michele Eniclerico from Penguin Random House, who were also instrumental in editing the book. I would also like to thank my brother Bobby Elijah Aviv and Giordona Aviv for their contributions to the Acid Watcher concepts.

I would like to thank Julia Serebrinsky for her multiple recipes pushing the envelope of the Acid Watcher ideas. In addition, I am very grateful to Giordona Aviv, chef Emiko Shimojo, and Maureen Schreyer for contributing some of the recipes as well. Special gratitude to dietitian Diane Insolia.

Many thanks go to my professional colleagues from my years at Columbia University: Drs. Andrew Blitzer, James Dillard, J. P. Mohr, Byron Thomashow, Lanny Close, Hector Rodriguez, Ian Storper, Henry Lodge, Herbert Pardes, and Steven Corwin. I am grateful to Florence and Herbert Irving for their largesse and vision, which enabled some of my original clinical research to be funded and carried out.

Much appreciation goes to Thomas Murry, SLP, PhD, the renowned speech-language pathologist who worked side by side with me for ten years at the Voice and Swallowing Center at Columbia. In addition, speech-language pathologists Eric Blicker, Manderly Cohen, Mark Berlin, Carolyn Gartner, Winston Cheng, Gaetano Fava, and Marta Kazandjian have continued to be extremely helpful in teaching and training endoscopy for swallowing. A special thanks to Drs. Steven Zeitels, Robert Sataloff, Robert Ossoff, Stanley Shapshay, Jamie Koufman, Peter Belafsky, Greg Postma, Blake Simpson, Milan Amin, Charles Ford, and Jeffrey Gallups, who were extraordinarily supportive of TNE from its infancy and ran enough interference to allow ideas off the beaten path to nurture and eventually flourish.

I would like to thank all my colleagues, staff, and administration at ENT and Allergy Associates, LLP—in particular, my fellow laryngologists at the Voice and Swallowing Center, Drs. David Godin, Jared Wasserman, Farhad Chowdhury, Joel Portnoy, Ajay Chitkara, Salvatore Taliercio, Philip Passalaqua, and Joseph DePietro, who have been instrumental in helping to broaden the breadth and depth of our Voice and Swallowing Center. I would also like to thank my partners in my clinical offices: Drs. Robert Green, Steven Sachs, Scott Markowitz, Guy Lin, Won Choe, Michael Bergstein, Jill Zeitlin, John County, and Lynelle Granady. Also, special thanks to Drs. Ofer Jacobowitz, Marc Levine, Moshe Ephrat, Lee Shangold, Krzysztof Nowak, and Lauren Zaretsky. Further thanks to the speech-language pathologists at ENT and Allergy Associates—Christie Block, Amanda Hembree, Danielle Falciglia, and Heather Jones—as well as my medical assistants, Cosette Osmani and Charleen Male. The administrative team at ENT and Allergy Associates, in particular Robert Glazer, Richard Effman, Jason Campbell, Nicole Monti, and Arthur Schwacke, were very helpful and encouraging.

Much gratitude to my medical colleagues around the country for their support: Drs. Ronny L. Jackson, James D'Orta, Dana Thompson, Marshall Strome, Michael Beninger, Seth Dailey, David Posner, Ken Altman, Eric Genden, Peak Woo, Mark Courey, Brett Miles, Michael Goldberg, Roger Crumley, Michael Pitman, Blair Jobe, and John Hunter.

The awareness of TNE overseas was greatly enhanced by Drs. Jean Abitbol, Gabriel Jaume, Manolo Tomas, Carmen Gorriz, Lance Maron, Sarmed Sami, Krish Ragunath, and Peter Friedland.

I would like to thank the following gastroenterologists for their support and guidance: Drs. Charles Lightdale, Lawrence Johnson, David Markowitz, Babak Mohajer, Jonathan LaPook, Stanley Benjamin, Phil Katz, Julian Abrams, Mark Pochapin, Arnon Lambroza, Joel Richter,

Acknowledgments

Lawrence Cohen, Reza Shaker, Alin Botoman, Michael Vaezi, Greg Haber, Robert Fath, Christopher DiMaio, David Greenwald, Gina Sam, Felice Schnoll-Sussman, Sharmila Anandasabapathy, Mark Noar, Nicholas Shaheen, David Katzka, Amitabh Chak, and Ashley Faulx.

Several stalwarts of the medical device industry and the food industry were critical in the transformation of ideas to reality, notably Lewis Pell, Katsumi Oneda, Nicholas Tsaclas, Ron Hadani, Mark Fletcher, Janis Saunier, David Damm, Ted Phelan, Alex Gorsky, Dr. Harlan Weisman, Bo Reilly, and Damion Michaels.

I am grateful to my friends and colleagues in the media and entertainment world who have brought attention to the dangers of untreated acid reflux, including Craig Kallman, Charlie Walk, Diane Sawyer, Dr. Mehmet Oz, Tim Sullivan, Dr. Michael Crupain, Steve Kroft, Jane Derenowski, Dr. Jay Adlersberg, Jane Brody, Carol Brody, Ian Axel, Alex Newell, Gad Elmaleh, Jen Kirkman, Gayle King, Chris Barron, John Turturro, and Jack Rosenthal.

Thank you to my close friends Jonathan Rapillo, Cherish Gallant, Robert Berman, Ira Kaufman, Herb Subin, Paul Michael Weiner, Jonathan Halpern, Jonathan Lowenberg, and Daniel Liebovici for their encouragement and support as this project developed and unfolded.

My appreciation and gratitude to Harvey Shapiro for his excellent legal advice as well as his continued friendship over the years.

A special thanks to my brother Oren Aviv for his support and encouragement, and my parents, Rena and David Aviv, for their everlasting love and faith in all of my medical endeavors since the beginning of my career, when I first put a Band-Aid on my mother's elbow when I was six.

Finally, I would like to thank my patients. I hope that by the writing of this book, I will continue to reach out to those in need, through the expression of the ideas set forth in this book.

281

Index

esophageal cancer, 4, 13, 15, 20–26, 29, 54, 59, 87, 105
 contributing factors to, 3–4, 47
 exercise and, 242–43
 forms of, *see* adenocarcinoma; squamous cell carcinoma
 GERD and, 41–43, 47
 obesity and, 41–43
 PPIs and, 64
 rates of, 3, 25–26, 105, 257, 259
esophageal sphincter, *see* lower esophageal sphincter; upper esophageal sphincter
esophagogastric junction, 26, 104
esophagus, 20–22, 23, 24, 43, 49–50, 58–62, 99, 108
 see also acid damage; acid reflux; acid reflux disease; esophageal cancer; heartburn; throatburn
exercise, 92, 114–15, 242–56, 258
 acid reflux and, 18, 242, 255–56
 consistency in, 244–45
 diet in combination with, 244
 esophageal cancer and, 242–43
 excess strain in, 249–50
 HIIT in, 251–55
 sleep and, 114–15, 243, 245
 timing of, 248–49

fats, dietary, 74–79
 see also saturated fats; trans fats; unsaturated fats
fennel, 132, 136, 137
 Sauté of Fennel, Red Cabbage, and Swiss Chard, 226–27
fermentation, 14, 74, 85, 109, 120
fiber, 7, 67, 69, 73, 81–82, 83–89, 126, 137, 138, 242
 in digestion, 81–84, 85, 86, 126
 food sources for, 89
 insoluble, 82–83
 soluble, 82
fibromyalgia, 258
fish, 133, 134, 135, 140
 Fish and Chips, 176–77
 Fresh Fish en Papillote with Potatoes, Olives, and Leeks, 224–25
 Miso-Agave-Glazed Halibut with Sesame Bok Choy, 174

omega-3 fats and, 77–78
 pH of, 94, 125, 153
 see also salmon
flavonoids, diabetes and, 37
FODMAP (fermentable, oligo-, di-, and monosaccharides, and polyols) carbohydrates, 74
fondue, Fruit Kabobs with Carob Fondue, 238
food:
 cravings for, *see* cravings
 fried, 78, 123, 130, 147
 low-fat, 68, 69, 72, 79, 108
 as medicine, 5, 43, 63, 136–39, 199
 preservatives in, 27–28, 30, 39, 80, 90, 109, 120, 123, 127, 130, 243
 processed, 14, 15, 16, 27, 28, 29, 30, 31, 39, 40, 43, 67, 71, 72, 76, 77, 78, 80, 86, 90, 95, 97–98, 108–9, 123, 124, 125, 130, 131, 144, 194, 243, 248, 257
Food and Drug Administration (FDA), 30
 Title 21 and, 27–28, 40
free radicals, 35–36, 38, 41, 43, 68, 97, 104, 123
Fresh Fish en Papillote with Potatoes, Olives, and Leeks, 224–25
Fresh Fruit, 165
fries, Cream of Broccoli Soup with Pepitas and Sweet Potato Fries, 185–86
frittata, Goat Cheese and Spinach Frittata, 207–8
fructans, 74, 122, 195
fruit, 88–89, 125, 127, 128, 135, 141, 125, 150–51, 197
 Fresh Fruit, 165
 Fruit Kabobs with Carob Fondue, 238
 Green Juice, 158–59
 Healthy Fruit-Flavored Yogurt #1, 204
 Healthy Fruit-Flavored Yogurt #2, 204
 see also specific fruit

gag reflex, 56
ganache:
 Poached Pears with Carob Ganache and Pistachios, 191–92
 Zucchini Muffins with "Chocolate" Ganache, 241
garlic, 96, 102, 122, 195

About the Author

Dr. Jonathan Aviv is the clinical director and founder of the Voice and Swallowing Center at ENT and Allergy Associates, LLP, in New York City. He is also clinical professor of otolaryngology, Icahn School of Medicine at Mount Sinai, and an attending physician at Mount Sinai Hospital in New York. Dr. Aviv is the former director of the Division of Head and Neck Surgery, Department of Otolaryngology—Head and Neck Surgery, College of Physicians and Surgeons, Columbia University.

He is the inventor and developer of the endoscopic air-pulse laryngeal sensory testing technology, known as FEESST. He also pioneered the development of awake, unsedated upper endoscopy, called transnasal esophagoscopy (TNE). Dr. Aviv has authored over sixty scientific papers in peer-reviewed journals and has written two medical textbooks, *Flexible Endoscopic Evaluation of Swallowing with Sensory Testing (FEESST)* and *Atlas of Transnasal Esophagoscopy.*

Dr. Aviv is past president of the American Broncho-Esophagological Association and the New York Laryngological Society, and former chairman of the Speech, Voice and Swallowing Disorders Committee, American Academy of Otolaryngology—Head and Neck Surgery.

Dr. Aviv has been in *New York Magazine*'s "Best Doctors" in 1998–2013 and 2015, *Best Doctors in America 2004–2015*, *Who's Who in America, Who's Who in Medicine and Healthcare,* and *Who's Who in Science and Engineering.*

Dr. Aviv has written blogs for the *Dr. Oz Show* website, Forbes .com, DysphagiaCafe.com, MindBodyGreen.com, and Livestrong.com, and has been featured in articles in the *New York Times* and the *Wall Street Journal*. He has also performed a TNE at the White House for Ronny L. Jackson, MD, physician to the president, and has appeared on *Good Morning America, The Dr. Oz Show, NBC Nightly News with Lester Holt,* CNN, *Inside Edition, Good Day New York, The Better Show,* Bloomberg Television, and the Discovery Channel.